EYE AND VISION RESEARCH DEVELOPMENTS

RETINOPATHY OF PREMATURITY (ROP)

CLASSIFICATION, RISK FACTORS AND TREATMENT

EYE AND VISION RESEARCH DEVELOPMENTS

Additional books in this series can be found on Nova's website under the Series tab.

Additional e-books in this series can be found on Nova's website under the e-book tab.

EYE AND VISION RESEARCH DEVELOPMENTS

RETINOPATHY OF PREMATURITY (ROP)

CLASSIFICATION, RISK FACTORS AND TREATMENT

ELMIRA AGUILAR
EDITOR

New York

Library of Congress Cataloging-in-Publication Data

ISBN: 978-1-63482-644-0
Library of Congress Control Number: 2015937446

Published by Nova Science Publishers, Inc. † New York

Contents

Preface

Retinopathy of prematurity is a disease caused by abnormal vessel regression of the retinal vasculature that affects premature infants with low birth weights. Despite significant improvements in screening guidelines and treatment modalties, ROP is still the leading cause of reversible paediatric blindness worldwide.

The authors of this book explore the possibility of applying the concept of fractal analysis to images of retinal blood vessels for morphometric analysis and classification; the quality of life for children with retinopathy of prematurity; the differences in ethnicity and socioeconomic status that influence the prevalence, risks, outcome and management of ROP; the outcome and prognostic factors of the intravitreal administration of bevacizumab for ROP; the outcomes of transpupillary diode laser photocoagulation for ROP; new therapeutic strategies for treating ROP and late complications that can develop and persistent into later childhood and even adult life (for example, long-term refractive errors, amblyopia, strabismus and optic nerve abnormalities)

Chapter 1 – Retinopathy of prematurity (ROP) is a hypoxia-induced neovascular retinal disease representing the major cause of blindness and visual impairment in children. Currently, surgical approaches (i.e. vitrectomy and laser photocoagulation) are the treatments of choice for ROP although they may result in a variety of complications, and new therapeutic strategies are eagerly required. In general, intravitreal injections of anti-vascular endothelial growth factor (VEGF) agents represent the most promising form of therapy to treat neovascular retinal disorders and there is expectancy for the use of these drugs to also treat ROP. However, for the use of these substances in ROP, the optimal choice of agent and dose remain unknown, while the possibility that the treatment may interfere with serum VEGF levels, and therefore affect normal vessel growth in developing tissues, remains to be considered. The serendipitous demonstration that a non-selective β-adrenergic receptor (β-AR) antagonist, propranolol, promotes the regression of infantile hemangiomas, the most common vascular tumor of infancy, aroused an interest around the involvement of the β-adrenergic system in angiogenic processes in humans. In particular, accumulating evidence indicates that the β-adrenergic system is involved in the hypoxia-induced neo-angiogenesis that is typically observed in ROP. In this respect, animal studies carried out in the mouse model of oxygen-induced retinopathy (OIR), which replicates the main features of ROP, have shown that β-AR blockade is effective in reducing pathological angiogenesis. For instance, propranolol has been demonstrated to inhibit hypoxia-induced VEGF expression and neo-angiogenesis when administered to OIR mice. Consequent to the encouraging results obtained in the animal model, a pilot clinical trial has shown that propranolol administered orally protects newborns from ROP progression. Indeed, compared to newborns with ROP stage 2 receiving standard treatment, the newborns with ROP stage 2 treated with oral propranolol showed a reduced progression to stage 3 or stage 3 plus and no newborns progressed to stage 4. However, some serious adverse effects of oral propranolol have been also reported. Therefore, this pilot study on the one hand has established the efficacy of propranolol treatment to counteract the progression of ROP, but on the other has indicated that the safety is a concern. Recent studies performed in rabbits have reported that the administration of propranolol through eye drops induces retinal concentrations of propranolol similar to those measured after oral administration, but with significantly lower plasma concentration. In addition, propranolol eye drops have been shown to reduce VEGF levels and retinal neovascularization in the mouse OIR model. These findings have opened the perspective of possible topical treatment with propranolol in newborns with ROP, and an ongoing study is indeed exploring the possibility of administering propranolol to newborns with ROP through eye drops with the objective to significantly reduce the side effects observed after oral propranolol administrations.

Chapter 2 – This text is focused on the area of quality of life for children with retinopathy of prematurity. It deals with retinopathy of prematurity and its influence on the personal experience of the quality of life in the pediatric population. The aim is to illustrate the diverse effects of retinopathy of prematurity on the quality of life of individuals and consequences related to it.

Scientific evaluation of the quality of life is currently phenomenon in the sphere of interest of many disciplines. Efforts to subjective assessment of quality of life is also currently enforced in special education. Quality of life could be characterized by several attributes, which illustrate the current state of scientific knowledge - broad applicability, multidimensional character, vague terminology definition, distinctive interdisciplinary, diverse interpretability, conceptual fragmentation and multifactorial conditionality. The suggested enumeration eloquently reflects the complexity, variability and lack of clarity of the concept of quality of life. Despite the diversity theoretical points, models, approaches and terminology, common element is conception of human as a bio-psycho-social complex. Emphasis is placed on subjective assessment and its preference before objectively measurable attributes. Given this fact is emerging a fundamental question - Why should be the quality of life actually explored? Spilker (1990) notes, that at the individual level, answer is obvious - the purpose is to improve individually oriented interventions. Comes to the fore the issue of the quality of life for specific client groups, the aim is an adequate level of support and optimization of complex interventions. In this context arose the concept of quality of life of children with retinopathy of prematurity. This disease remains the leading cause of childhood blindness in developed and moderately developed countries. Thanks to this is ROP in interest of ophthalmologists worldwide. ROP causes up to 70% of pediatric blindness (Kuchynka et al. 2007). This vazoproliferative retinal disease mainly affects premature infants with low birth weight. Its incidence increases with a percentage of surviving of extremely preterm infants. The spectrum of the resulting anatomical and structural changes and functional consequences is variable, but almost always impaired visual function as a result. New possibilities of therapy with bevacizumab have encouraging results, however ROP and especially its atypical forms remain the focus of experts. Is clear that the ROP plays an essential role in the development of visual functions - affects early critical period of visual development and is located at key post - on the retina. Even in cases where the ROP regresses spontaneously, there are certain anatomical changes that can secondarily cause visual impairment. Current scientific and technical progress in medical care, respectively neonatology, perinatology, and especially ophthalmology, significantly improved the prognosis of visual function, even though ROP may have fatal consequences in the form of complete loss of visual perception. As part of our research, we tried to identify and describe some of the attributes that can specifically determine the quality of life of each individual. Some of the effects of visual impairment can hamper life satisfaction and well-being and may affect the fundamental pillars of quality of life. ROP thus remains the current medical, social, economic and ethical issue. The aim of qualitatively oriented research was the identification and comprehensive analysis of the specifics of the target group and their depth description. The aim is to optimize intervention process and ideally improve the quality of life of clients. The basic idea is the subjective evaluation of the impact of ROP on the quality of life of the child. One of the objectives of this work is to identify the relevant indicators of quality of life specific to the child population with this type of visual impairment. In the text is presented theoretical background which make comprehensive theoretical framework for design research. Subsequently are presented outcomes of empirical research, which take the form of primary probe into the selected area.

Chapter 3 – Retinopathy of prematurity is a disease caused by abnormal vessel regression of the retinal vasculature that affects premature infants with low birth weights. This paper explores the possibility of applying the concept of fractal analysis to images of retinal blood vessels for morphometric analysis and classification. More than 100 neonates were screening with RetCam 3 device by the experienced ophthalmologist who chose 101 suitable images and set them into three groups, according to the presence of the ROP and the stage of ROP development. Black and white binary images were carried out by box dimension quantifying the space-filling, shape and tortuosity of retinal blood vessels. Accordingly, grey-scale images were investigated by the lacunar and multifractal analysis, which quantifies heterogeneity and multifractal spectra, respectively. The results indicate that the gestational age of premature births did not influence the box dimension, homogeneity and multifractal spectra. The blood vessels in the retinae with severe retinopathy of prematurity are more heterogeneous, complex and have a higher degree of vessel aberration than those vessels with infants without retinopathy. Multifractal analysis, however, did show significant differences between only between those two stages of the retinopathy. The authors have demonstrated that objective parameters for morphometric analysis and classifying of retinopathy can be found by applying the fractal and multifractal analyses. The next step in developing might be to establish a clinical standard based on fractal and multifractal measures. Another application could be the development of software that can be implemented in standard ophthalmologic imaging.

Chapter 4 – Retinopathy of prematurity (ROP) is a vaso-proliferative disease targeting the developing retina particularly in those with low birth weight and preterm gestation. Despite significant improvements in screening guidelines and treatment modalities, ROP is still the leading cause of reversible paediatric blindness worldwide. The 1984 Classification of Retinopathy of Prematurity and the 1988 Cyrotherapy for ROP (CRYO-ROP) study made screening for ROP imperative and subsequently improved the visual prognosis of this condition. The aim of screening is to detect infants with ROP and to deliver treatment in a timely manner to prevent irreversible visual loss. With advancements in the field of neonatology, smaller and sicker infants are surviving and therefore ROP continues to be a growing medical and public concern. Differences in ethnicity and socioeconomic status influence the prevalence, risks, outcome, and management of ROP. In this chapter, the incidences, risk factors, screening guidelines, and treatment trends will be reviewed and the characteristics in various preterm subtypes (extremely low birth weight, extremely preterm, multiple pregnancies, and co-twins) will also be highlighted with reference to their risks in ROP development.

Chapter 5 – Purpose: The purpose of this study is to evaluate the outcomes of transpupillary diode laser photocoagulation for retinopathy of prematurity (ROP) in the authors' hospital. *Methods:* This is a retrospective case series that was carried out at the "Iuliu Hatieganu" University of Medicine and Pharmacy from Cluj-Napoca, Romania. The records of all the infants who received indirect diode laser photocoagulation for ROP, between January 1st 2006 – October 31st 2014 were reviewed. The following parameters were analized: gestational age, birth weight, postmenstrual age at treatment, postnatal age at treatment, type of pregnancy (unique or multiple), gender, number of laser sessions, ROP classification (zone and stage of the disease), postlaser evolution (regression or progression of ROP). The statistical analysis was performed with the program SPSS 22.0. *Results*: During the above mentioned period of time, the authors performed diode laser photocoagulation for ROP in 168 eyes of 87 infants: 48 males (55.20%) and 39 females (44.80%). Gestational age was between 24 and 33 weeks (mean 28.67 weeks ± 2 weeks SD) and birth weight was between 600 and 1700 grams (mean 1123.33 grams ± 276.41grams SD). The postnatal age at treatment was between 5 and 13 weeks (mean 8.41weeks ± 1.97 weeks SD) and the postmenstrual age at treatment was between 32 and 41weeks (mean 37.10 weeks ± 1.77 weeks SD). We classified the 168 treated eyes into two categories: classic disease (stage 3+ ROP in zones 1 or 2) – 138 eyes (82.14%) and aggressive posterior ROP (AP-ROP) – 30 eyes (17.85%). ROP regressed in 148 eyes (88.09%). The success rate was significantly better in the classic ROP (95.65%) as compared to AP-ROP (53.33%). *Discussion*: The rationale for the use of laser in ROP is discussed. The factors that influenced the ROP regression are analyzed, as follows: individual factors (ROP category, birth weight, gestational age, type of pregnancy, sex of the infant), timing of the laser treatment (postmenstrual age, postnatal age). *Conclusion:* Indirect diode laser photocoagulation proved its efficacy in the treatment of ROP: in 88.58% of the treated eyes ROP regressed and the retina remained attached.

Chapter 6 – Retinopathy of prematurity is a lifelong disease. Compared to full term population, higher prevalence of refractive errors, amblyopia, stabismus, reduction in visual field, impaired color vision and contrast sensitivity is found. Preterm delivery resulted in a disrupted development of both anterior and posterior segment of the eye. Preterm birth showed a significant impact on axial length, keratometry values, corneal thickness, lower and higher order refractive errors of the cornea. The anterior segment parameters such as shallower anterior chamber depth and thicker lens were determined by the presence of retinopathy in the acute phase. In the posterior segment, higher foveal thickness was found compared to full-term subjects. The impairment of normal centrifugal movement of foveal cone nuclei and inner retinal cells is supposed. Pigment disturbances, macular dragging due to regressed retinopathy in the periphery, developmental restriction of optic nerve head, thinner choroid are associated with worse best corrected visual acuity in formerly preterm patient. Due to the peripheral degenerative changes in the retina, abnormal vitreoretinal interface, retinal detachment either rhegmatogeneous or tractional can develop not only in acute phase of ROP but in the late adulthood, as well.

Chapter 7 – *Background*: In this chapter the authors aim to evaluate the outcome and prognostic factors of the intravitreal administration of bevacizumab for retinopathy of prematurity (ROP), as monotherapy and associated with laser treatment, as emerged from our experience. *Methods*: This is a retrospective case series that was carried out at the "Iuliu Hatieganu" University of Medicine and Pharmacy from Cluj-Napoca, Romania. It includes all the consecutive infants who received intravitreal bevacizumab for ROP, between January 1st 2009 and December 31st 2013. The following data were recorded: birth weight, gestational age, gender, type of pregnancy (unique or multiple), timing (postmenstrual age and postnatal age at treatment), immediate result (ROP regression or progression), late ROP recurrence (52 weeks after treatment), the necessity of laser. The statistical analysis was performed with the program SPSS 22.0. *Results:* The study includes 97 eyes of 49 infants. According to the number of eyes, 60 had aggressive posterior ROP (61.85%), 15 had bilateral zone I stage 3+ ROP (30.61%), one had unilateral zone I stage 3+ ROP (2.04%), 2 had bilateral stage IV A ROP (4.08%) and one had in one eye zone I stage 3+ ROP and in the fellow eye, stage IV A ROP (2.04%). One week after the bevacizumab injection, ROP regressed in 83 eyes (85.56%). Discussion: The place of anti-VEGF treatment in ROP is emphasized. The advantages of anti-VEGF as compared to laser are discussed, but also the possible systemic and local complications associated with this therapy. The factors that influenced the outcomes of anti-VEGF treatment are analyzed according to the statistical data. *Conclusion:* ROP regression rate after the intravitreal administration of bevacizumab monotherapy was 85.56% in the authors' series.

In: Retinopathy of Prematurity (ROP)
Editor: Elmira Aguilar
ISBN: 978-1-63482-644-0

Chapter 1

Targeting the Beta-Adrenergic System to Treat Retinopathy of Prematurity: A New Therapeutic Approach?

Luca Filippi[1,*], Maurizio Cammalleri[2,†] and Massimo Dal Monte[2,‡]

[1]Neonatal Intensive Care Unit, Medical Surgical Fetal-neonatal Department, 'A. Meyer' University Children's Hospital, Florence, Italy

[2]Department of Biology, Unit of General Physiology, University of Pisa, Italy

Abstract

Retinopathy of prematurity (ROP) is a hypoxia-induced neovascular retinal disease representing the major cause of blindness and visual impairment in children. Currently, surgical approaches (i.e. vitrectomy and laser photocoagulation) are the treatments of choice for ROP

* Email: luca.filippi@meyer.it.

† Email: maurizio.cammalleri@unipi.it.

‡ Corresponding Author: Massimo Dal Monte, Department of Biology, University of Pisa, via San Zeno, 31-56127 Pisa (Italy). Email: massimo.dalmonte@unipi.it.

although they may result in a variety of complications, and new therapeutic strategies are eagerly required. In general, intravitreal injections of anti-vascular endothelial growth factor (VEGF) agents represent the most promising form of therapy to treat neovascular retinal disorders and there is expectancy for the use of these drugs to also treat ROP. However, for the use of these substances in ROP, the optimal choice of agent and dose remain unknown, while the possibility that the treatment may interfere with serum VEGF levels, and therefore affect normal vessel growth in developing tissues, remains to be considered. The serendipitous demonstration that a non-selective β-adrenergic receptor (β-AR) antagonist, propranolol, promotes the regression of infantile hemangiomas, the most common vascular tumor of infancy, aroused an interest around the involvement of the β-adrenergic system in angiogenic processes in humans. In particular, accumulating evidence indicates that the β-adrenergic system is involved in the hypoxia-induced neo-angiogenesis that is typically observed in ROP. In this respect, animal studies carried out in the mouse model of oxygen-induced retinopathy (OIR), which replicates the main features of ROP, have shown that β-AR blockade is effective in reducing pathological angiogenesis. For instance, propranolol has been demonstrated to inhibit hypoxia-induced VEGF expression and neo-angiogenesis when administered to OIR mice. Consequent to the encouraging results obtained in the animal model, a pilot clinical trial has shown that propranolol administered orally protects newborns from ROP progression. Indeed, compared to newborns with ROP stage 2 receiving standard treatment, the newborns with ROP stage 2 treated with oral propranolol showed a reduced progression to stage 3 or stage 3 plus and no newborns progressed to stage 4. However, some serious adverse effects of oral propranolol have been also reported. Therefore, this pilot study on the one hand has established the efficacy of propranolol treatment to counteract the progression of ROP, but on the other has indicated that the safety is a concern. Recent studies performed in rabbits have reported that the administration of propranolol through eye drops induces retinal concentrations of propranolol similar to those measured after oral administration, but with significantly lower plasma concentration. In addition, propranolol eye drops have been shown to reduce VEGF levels and retinal neovascularization in the mouse OIR model. These findings have opened the perspective of possible topical treatment with propranolol in newborns with ROP, and an ongoing study is indeed exploring the possibility of administering propranolol to newborns with ROP through eye drops with the objective to significantly reduce the side effects observed after oral propranolol administrations.

Introduction

Retinopathy of prematurity (ROP) is a neovascular retinal disease characterized by leakage and/or neovascularization from retinal vessels of the inner retina causing damage to retinal tissue and impaired visual function. The incidence of ROP is closely correlated with the weight and the gestational age at birth. Despite current therapies, ROP continues to be a highly debilitating disease, representing the major cause of blindness and visual impairment in children.

Ablation of non-vascularized retina by cryotherapy was emerged in the 1980s as a method to reduce structural and functional disease associated to ROP [1]. In the CRYO-ROP study, preterm newborns with stage 3 ROP in zone 1 or 2 in the presence of "plus" disease were subjected to transscleral cryotherapy in one randomly selected eye, while the other eye remained untreated and served as a control [2]. The evaluation of outcomes at 10 years after treatment showed that eyes treated with cryotherapy were much less likely than control eyes to be blind [3]. Despite the efficacy of cryotherapy in treating ROP, several drawbacks prompted investigators to pursue other treatment modalities. For instance, cryotherapy may be easily administered to anterior locations, but posterior treatment is more difficult and often requires conjunctival incisions.

In more recent years, the choice of treatment for ROP has shifted from cryotherapy to diode laser photocoagulation after clinical studies showing the superiority of laser therapy to cryotherapy [4, 5] and laser photocoagulation of the peripheral avascular retina is currently the gold standard in the therapy of ROP. Over time, the timing of treatment has moved to an earlier stage of the disease but, despite the advances, progression to retinal detachment occurs in 12% of eyes [6]. Additionally, laser therapy has some disadvantages including intraocular hemorrhage, cataract formation, and significant decrease in peripheral vision due to ablation of peripheral retina.

Aggressive posterior ROP (AP-ROP) is a severe form of ROP characterized by posterior location (zone I or posterior zone II), severe plus disease, and a rapidly progressive course [7]. Management of AP-ROP is difficult and often associated with retinal detachment despite laser or cryotherapy treatment [1, 6]. Therefore, vitrectomy may be considered as an alternative to treat AP-ROP and severe ROP (stage 4 and 5) in eyes that progress to retinal detachment, although it results in generally poor outcomes.

The process of neovascularization is stimulated by proangiogenic growth factors, particularly vascular endothelial growth factor (VEGF), therefore the use of intravitreally injected anti-VEGF agents, approved by Food and Drug Administration for the treatment of some ocular neovascular diseases in adults, has been regarded as an interesting pharmacological approach to the management of ROP. However, limitations of the use of intravitreal injections of anti VEGF agents are evident in the treatment of ROP. In this respect, the larger concerns are related to whether the anti-VEGF compounds act systemically and are damaging to the immature retina. Indeed, while the use of anti-VEGF therapies may appear as an attractive alternative to laser ablation, the optimal choice of agent and dose remains uncertain, and suppression of serum VEGF levels might interfere with the processes of normal angiogenesis in the developing tissues [8]. In a recent study using a mouse model of ROP, inhibition of VEGF in developing eyes has been found to delay vascular growth in the short-term, but to induce functional decrease in the long-term with persistent changes in neural retinal structures [9].

New pharmacological treatments, including gene therapy [10, 11] and supplementation with omega-3 fatty acids or IGF-1 [12-14] also represent interesting pharmacological approaches to the management of ROP. In this line, an extension of the therapeutic arsenal with the identification of new pharmacologic targets is needed to improve the efficacy and the safety of the treatments. The β-adrenergic system may represent one of these new targets. In this chapter, we gather evidence of the involvement of the β-adrenergic system in retinal pathologies characterized by aberrant growth of neovessels to evaluate the proposal of the possible use of β-adrenergic drugs in the clinics. To this aim, we first provide an overview of the pathogenesis of ROP and of animal models recapitulating the main aspects of the pathophysiology of this disease.

Pathogenesis of ROP

ROP is a retinal neovascular disease of developmental origin [15]. In humans, retinal vascularization is completed at the time of birth, therefore the process of normal vascular development can be disrupted in preterm newborns and this may lead to retinal neovascularization. From a clinical point of view, pathophysiology of ROP is characterized by two phases, a first vaso-obliterative phase and a second vaso-proliferative phase.

After birth, preterm newborns move from the *in utero* environment, characterized by a pO_2 of about 35 mmHg, to the relative hyperoxia of the extrauterine environment (pO_2 of about 55-80 mmHg), and this relative hyperoxia may be worsened by supplemental oxygen therapy [16]. During this phase, the expression of hypoxia-induced proangiogenic factors, including VEGF, is down-regulated, promoting the arrest or retardation of the growth of existing retinal blood vessels. In addition, already formed vessels constrict and retract. As the newborn matures, the increase in metabolic requirements of the developing retina, in the absence of an appropriate vascularization, leads to tissue hypoxia. The first phase of ROP occurs from birth to postmenstrual age approximately 30-32 weeks [17].

The second phase of ROP is characterized by the vaso-proliferative phase of compensatory, often uncontrolled, neovascularization and begins around 32-34 weeks postmenstrual age. New vessels form at the junction between the vascularized retina and the avascular area. These new vessels, due to inappropriate development and patterning, cannot sufficiently oxygenate the retina and can bleed easily. Over time, this uncontrolled vessel growth produces a fibrous scar extending from the retina to the vitreous whose retraction may lead to retinal detachment and likely blindness [18].

The alternation of a hyperoxic and a hypoxic phase in neonatal retina with subsequent neovascularization has been used to generate animal models of ischemic retinopathy, which recapitulate the pathophysiology of ROP.

Animal Models of ROP

The major models used to study ROP are the animal models of oxygen-induced retinopathy (OIR). The OIR model was first developed in cat [19]. Then, this model has been also developed in rat [20], mouse [21], dog [22], and zebrafish [23]. The different models have in common the same mechanism: exposure to hyperoxia, which leads to vaso-oblietration, and return to normoxia (experienced as relative hypoxia) or to moderate hypoxia, leading to neovascularization. Neovascularization occurs at the junction between the vascularized and nonvascularized retina, followed by normalization of the vascular pattern with regression of the abnormal vessels in mice [21]. Retinal detachment that can be seen in the late stage of ROP occurs in the dog OIR model, but not in the mouse or cat OIR model [24, 25].

The Mouse OIR Model

The most widely used model of ROP is the mouse OIR model. The main advantage of this model is the possible use of genetic manipulation, as transgenic mice can be used to directly study the roles of different genes on pathological neovascularization. Other advantages are the reproducibility of the model and a reliable method of quantifying retinal neovascularization [26]. A major disadvantage of this model is the fact that in mice, in contrast to humans, the central retinal vessels, rather than the peripheral ones, are obliterated during exposure to hyperoxia. Despite this difference, the mouse OIR model very closely recapitulates the pathologic events occurring during ischemia-induced neovascularization [27]. In the original model [21], C57BL/6J mouse pups and their nursing mothers are placed in 75% oxygen from postnatal day 7 (PD7) to PD12. During this hyperoxic phase, vasoconstriction and regression of immature capillaries in the central retina occur, with maximum vaso-obliteration reached at about PD9. The extension of the central avascular area regresses from PD9 to PD12, possibly as a consequence of the increasing metabolic demand of the developing retina [28-30]. At PD12, mice are returned to room air, which is experienced as relative hypoxia. As a consequence, stabilization of the α subunit of the transcription factor hypoxia-inducible factor 1 (HIF-1α) occurs, followed by the up-regulation of HIF-1-dependent genes, including those of proangiogenic factors such as VEGF [30, 31]. In this phase, proangiogenic factors induce both revascularization of the central avascular area and pathological neovascularization. Newly formed retinal vessels grow from the retinal surface towards the vitreous and generate preretinal tufts, that is small caliber unorganized vessels prone to leakage which are similar to pathological vessels seen in human ROP [21]. The growth of neovessels peaks at PD17, a time characterized by the maximum extent of pathological neovascularization and plasma leakage. From PD17, neovascularization begins to regress and at PD25 both the neovascular tufts and the central avascular area are almost disappeared [32].

In mice, different severities of OIR have been found to develop in different strains. For instance, C57BL/6J mice show relatively lower production of proangiogenic factors than 129S3/SvIM mice [33]. Noteworthy, some strains of mice, such as BALB/cByJ, do not develop pathological neovascularization at all, despite hyperoxia-induced vascular obliteration [34].

Using the OIR model in C57BL/6J mice, we have evidenced a role of the β-adrenergic system in retinal neovascular pathology, supporting the possibility that drugs targeting β-adrenergic receptors (β-ARs) may have a therapeutic potential. These results have prompted an interest in exploring the possibility that the administration of β-AR blockers, such as propranolol, a β1/β2-AR antagonist, may help in the treatment of ROP. Before reviewing the experimental studies addressing these issues, we will explain the rationale that led us to investigate this possibility. Then we will provide some basic information on the β-adrenergic system in the mammalian retina, which will serve as a background for the evaluation of the involvement of this system in retinal pathologies, investigated in animal studies as well as in clinical trials.

A Rationale to Investigate the Potential of β-AR Blockers in Reducing Retinal Angiogenesis

The most solid background for the study of the role of β-ARs in retinal neovascular pathologies is represented by recent studies demonstrating the efficacy of propranolol in the treatment of infantile hemangiomas, the most frequent benign tumors in infancy. They are tumors of endothelial cells and affect 5-10% of all newborns, with a significantly higher incidence (up to 30%) in premature newborns [35]. It normally undergoes a gradual reduction to resolve by the age of 5. In infantile hemangiomas, neovascularization is driven by increased levels of HIF-1 [36] and of VEGF [37]. Since 2008, a large number of studies have reported the unexpected rapid regression of infantile hemangiomas in newborns treated with propranolol [38, 39] to the point that propranolol has become the treatment of choice for complicated infantile hemangiomas. The efficacy of this treatment has been explained on the basis that β2-AR blockade inhibits the production of VEGF. Indeed, VEGF expression in hemangioma-derived endothelial cells has been reported to be down-regulated by propranolol in a dose-dependent manner [40] through a HIF-1-mediated mechanism [41].

The information obtained in these studies constitutes a strong rationale for investigations on the involvement of the β-adrenergic system in neovascular retinal pathologies and for the possible exploitation of drugs targeting this system as possible new therapies.

The β-Adrenergic System in the Retina

The β-adrenergic system is part of the sympathetic autonomic nervous system and it is composed of three different receptors, β1-, β2- and β3-ARs, and their ligands, epinephrine (E) and norepinephrine (NE).

The expression of β-ARs in the retina is well documented [42], although their exact localization has not been fully clarified yet. β1-ARs are primarily expressed by Müller cells, the principal glial cells of the retina [43], and by endothelial cells [44, 45]. β2-ARs constitute the most variegated β-AR subtype, as they seem to be expressed by multiple retinal cell types including Müller cells and, likely, different populations of retinal neurons [43, 46, 47]. β3-ARs seem to be expressed only by blood vessels, probably by endothelial cells [44, 47, 48].

The source of E and NE in the retina is incompletely understood. It is likely that most of the NE released in the rat retina is associated with sympathetic nerve terminals and that E is contained in intrinsic retinal cells. Indeed, retinal sympathectomy decreases the retinal concentration of NE but has no effect on that of E [49]. The sympathetic innervations mainly controls the choroidal circulation, while retinal circulation lacks autonomic innervation and is mainly regulated by local factors [50]. Therefore, NE seems to reach the retina coming from sympathetic terminals innervating the choroidal vessels. On the other hand, there is also evidence that NE may be produced by amacrine cells and ganglion cells [51-53]. In addition, the enzyme converting dopamine to NE, dopamine β hydroxylase, has been localized to photoreceptors and in the outer plexiform, inner plexiform and ganglion cell layers [54]. An additional source of E and/or NE in hypoxic conditions may be represented by the endothelial cells of retinal vessels if they behavior is similar to that of bovine aorta endothelial cells. Indeed, it has been reported that bovine aorta endothelial cells contain the enzymes for E and NE synthesis and that under hypoxic conditions they overexpress catecholamines [55].

Role of the β-Adrenergic System in OIR

In the last few years, we have performed a series of investigations using the OIR model in the C57BL/6J mouse strain. As a result of our studies, we have found that the pathological angiogenesis that typically develops in this model is sustained, at least in part, by increased β-adrenergic transmission.

Indeed, we have observed that in OIR mice retinal levels of NE are almost doubled in comparison to control mice [56]. This finding is in line with previous observations in the rat brain [57-58] and suggests that increased levels of NE may, in turn, overstimulate β-ARs and potentially activate signaling pathways leading to the growth of new retinal vessels. In this respect, alterations of sympathetic transmission are known to contribute to the development of vascular abnormalities in diabetic retinopathy [59-61]. These findings, together, indicate a crucial role of the sympathetic system in regulating retinal angiogenesis and suggest that drugs that can restore sympathetic homeostasis could effectively ameliorate vascular dysfunctions in OIR mice.

Propranolol Reduces Retinal Neovascularization in OIR

The angiogenic switch represented by β-ARs may be inhibited by β-AR blockade, in particular by β2-AR blockade, as indicated by our studies [46, 48]. In this respect, systemic administrations of propranolol, a β1/β2-AR blocker, to OIR mice from PD12 to PD16 reduce retinal expression of both VEGF and insulin-like growth factor (IGF)-1, the formation of neovascular tufts, and vascular leakage due to blood-retinal barrier (BRB) breakdown [48]. The role of VEGF in inducing damage to tight junction proteins leading to vascular leakage from BRB has been well established [62], therefore the amelioration in BRB breakdown induced by propranolol is likely to be mediated by reduction of VEGF expression. Noteworthy, although IGF-1 has been described as a potent inducer of VEGF [63], the propranolol-induced inhibitions of IGF-1 and of VEGF seem to constitute two independent events that run in parallel [48]. However, since IGF-1 is required to promote VEGF activation of vascular endothelial cell proliferation and survival [64], propranolol may affect retinal angiogenesis both directly, by decreasing the angiogenic effect of VEGF, and indirectly, by inhibiting the permissive action of IGF-1. The decrease in VEGF up-regulation induced by propranolol in the retina of OIR mice is not observed when propranolol is administered to control mice, suggesting different patterns of regulation of VEGF expression in normoxic and hypoxic conditions [48]. Most importantly, these observations suggest that β-AR blockade induced by propranolol administration only affects the VEGF production promoted by hypoxia, and probably mediated by HIF-1. The finding that propranolol partially prevents the stabilization of HIF-1α, which is greatly enhanced in the retina of OIR mice, strengthens this hypothesis, indicating that HIF-1 is likely to participate in the mechanisms coupling β1/β2-AR blockade to the inhibition of VEGF expression [48]. In this respect, carvedilol, a nonselective β-AR blocker, reduces the expression of both HIF-1α and VEGF in a rat model of cardiac hypertrophy [65]. In addition, in the retina of OIR mice, statins exert beneficial effects in ameliorating vascular dysfunction by preventing hypoxia-induced HIF-1α stabilization [66]. Our results obtained in OIR mice are consistent with those reported in the retina of OIR rats, where the non-selective β1/β2-AR antagonist timolol has been observed to induce VEGF down-regulation and to diminish the severity of retinal neovascularization [67-69].

The effects of propranolol against angiogenesis in OIR mice has been confirmed by clinical data demonstrating that, in patients with age-related macular degeneration (AMD), propranolol reduces the need for repeated intravitreal injections of bevacizumab [70]. In addition, in a mouse model of choroidal neovascularization, which is a model of wet AMD, intraperitoneal injections of propranolol result in a 50% reduction in angiogenesis, demonstrating that β-AR blockade induces a strong inhibitory effect on the extent of choroidal neovascularization in this model [71].

In order to perform a translational approach in light of a possible use of propranolol as a therapeutic against ROP, the topical application of propranolol to OIR mice has been considered. Indeed, systemic administration of propranolol may have potential adverse effects in newborns including bradycardia, hypotension, and hypoglycemia [72]. In this respect, topical application of propranolol may be more selective in comparison with systemic administration since the drug is delivered directly to the target tissues, minimizing systemic exposure and reducing undesirable systemic effects. In a recent study, the effects of propranolol applied as eye drops on retinal angiogenesis in OIR mice have been investigated. Propranolol, applied on the eye surface from PD12 to PD16, efficiently reaches the retina where it can be recovered at concentrations in the order of micrograms per gram of retinal tissue, indicating that the drug is taken up by the tissue from the administration site and is conveyed to the posterior segment of the eye [73]. Most importantly, 2% propranolol eye drops inhibit the effects of hypoxia in the retina of OIR mice with results similar to those observed after systemic administration [48], that is reduction of hypoxia-induced up-regulation of angiogenic molecules and of associated transcription factors and inhibition of neovascular tuft formation [73]. Noteworthy propranolol effects on retinal neovascularization can still be detected at PD 21, when spontaneous regression of neovascularization and reduction of the avascular areas are observed [28], indicating that propranolol administration between PD12 and PD16, the period at which hypoxia triggers the maximal response, may be critical to obtain long lasting effects. These data suggest that eye drop administration may represent a possible valid route to secure propranolol delivery to the retina to counteract neovascular pathologies minimizing systemic exposure and avoiding side effects. In this respect, a pharmacokinetic study aimed at identifying the most appropriate concentration of propranolol eye drops capable to give a more favorable retina/plasma ratio compared with oral administration has been performed in rabbits [74]. The comparison between the pharmacokinetic results obtained in rabbits receiving oral propranolol eye drops show that topical chronic administration of 0.1% propranolol results in retinal concentrations of the drug comparable with those obtained after oral chronic administration of propranolol at 1mg/kg/day. In addition, plasma levels after topical propranolol are about 10–20 times lower than after oral drug administration, suggesting a better retinal/plasma ratio for eye drops. In addition, 0.1% propranolol-based eye drops are safe and do not alter ocular structures, as demonstrated by Draize test and histological investigations performed in propranolol-treated rabbits.

Results obtained in propranolol-treated OIR C57BL/6J mice indicate that propranolol is effective in counteracting retinal pathological neovascularization. On the other hand, a study performed in an OIR mouse model based on a different strain (129S6 mice), reports that propranolol fails to suppress retinal neovascularization or up-regulation of growth factors, including VEGF [75]. The different genetic background of the mice may have contributed to the different responses of the retina to hypoxia [76]. For instance, the 129S6 mouse strain seems to have a more robust neovascular response compared to the C57BL/6J strain [77]. In this respect, it is worth mentioning that a wide variability exists in clinical expression of ROP between non-African American and African American newborns [78], and that this variability is apparently due to polymorphisms of intracellular effectors linked to β-AR function, that have been reported in many African American people [79]. In addition, β-AR gene variants seem to influence cardiac responses to β-AR agonists in patients on β-AR blocker therapy [80]. Besides the difference in genetic background, a dramatic up-regulation of β3-ARs has been reported in the OIR 129S6 mouse model [75], which may also play a role in the different response of OIR C57BL/6J and 129S6 mice to propranolol (see below). The same study using 129S6 mice also reported that propranolol is unable to suppress human retinal microvascular endothelial cell proliferation, unless at high, non-physiological concentrations [75], and these data were discussed as an evidence of the lack of propranolol efficacy in contrasting retinal neovascularization. In effect, if we consider that β2-ARs are mostly implicated in the response to propranolol, as observed in the experiments with C57BL/6J mice (see below), this result is not surprising, since only β1-ARs and β3-ARs (but not β2-ARs) appear to be expressed by human retinal endothelial cells [44].

Role of β2-ARs in OIR

To better define the role of the β-adrenergic system in the neovascular retinal response in C57BL/6J mice, the involvement of specific β-AR subtypes has been investigated employing selective β1- or β2-AR blockers. Subcutaneous administrations to OIR C57BL/6J mice of ICI 118, 551, a selective β2-AR blocker, decrease retinal levels of proangiogenic factors similar to propranolol [48] and reduce pathological neovascularization [46], suggesting that activation of β2-ARs constitutes an important part of the retinal response to hypoxia. Interestingly, Müller glial cells, which in the mouse retina are known to express VEGF under hypoxic conditions [81], are also likely to express β2-ARs [46], suggesting the possibility that β2-ARs play a role in directly regulating VEGF expression and/or release by these cells. In addition to decreasing neovascularization, β2-AR blockade with ICI 118,551 is also effective in ameliorating electroretinographic responses, which are affected in OIR mice [46], indicating that β2-AR signaling in the OIR retina not only plays a pro-angiogenic action, but is also responsible for direct or indirect functional damage. Atenolol, mainly a β1-AR blocker [82], does not affect retinal levels of proangiogenic factors and pathological neovascularization in OIR mice [46]. This seems to exclude a role of β1-ARs in the regulation of retinal angiogenesis in hypoxic conditions. A similar conclusion comes from studies in a rat model of diabetic retinopathy, where atenolol is unable to improve either electroretinographic responses [83] or vascular pathological changes [84], or from studies in human retinal endothelial cells, where xamoterol, a β1-AR partial agonist, is ineffective in inducing proliferation or migration of these cells [44].

Together, our findings indicate that in OIR mice the angiogenic switch represented by β-AR stimulation secondary to increased levels of NE would be inhibited by the blockade of β2-ARs. However, treatment of OIR mice with systemic administrations of isoproterenol, a classical nonselective β-AR agonist, surprisingly results in significantly decreased retinal VEGF levels and reduced pathological neovascularization [56]. This unexpected result was explained by the observations that isoproterenol reduces the levels of membrane-associated β2-ARs without affecting those of β1- and β3-ARs, suggesting down-regulation of β2-ARs caused by prolonged agonist exposure, and decreases adenylylcyclase activity, indicating a decrease of the efficiency of β-AR coupling mechanisms [56]. Thus, the antiangiogenic effects of isoproterenol are likely to be due to β2-AR desensitization caused by excessive stimulation. Indeed, β2-AR down-regulation after isoproterenol has been reported in different experimental models [85-87] and appears to be a key component of prolonged agonist-induced receptor desensitization. In general, uncoupling between G protein-coupled receptors and G proteins depends on receptor phosphorylation operated by kinases such as G-protein receptor coupled kinases (GRKs) [88]. Among them, GRK2, which is expressed in the mouse retina [89], is the prototype GRK for β-AR desensitization [90] and is known to act at β2-ARs [91, 92]. The expression of GRK2 is increased in the retina of OIR mice after treatment with isoproterenol [56], suggesting that β-AR agonism may promote GRK2-mediated β2-AR phosphorylation and, in turn, β2-AR uncoupling from G proteins. The isoproterenol-induced desensitization of β2-ARs in OIR retinas is further suggested by the observation that β-arrestin 2, which is involved in desensitization of β2-ARs [93], increases its recruitment to β2-ARs in the presence of isoproterenol [56].

In summary, results from studies using propranolol or isoproterenol indicate that reduction in β2-AR signaling may counteract hypoxia-induced angiogenic processes in the retina of OIR mice. This suggests that maintaining β2-AR signaling homeostasis is crucial to counteract vascular abnormalities and that sympathetic β-adrenergic transmission may represent a target for therapeutic intervention against retinal vascular pathologies. In proceeding further in the characterization of the β-adrenergic system in the OIR mouse model, our studies have highlighted the role of another subtype of β-ARs, the β3-AR, in regulating retinal angiogenesis in OIR C57BL/6J mice.

Role of β3-ARs in Retinal Angiogenesis

After the classical distinction between β1- and β2-AR subtypes [94], in the 1980s the β-AR family has been formally enriched with a third β-AR, called β3-AR, cloned in humans in 1989 and initially identified in adipose tissue [95]. More recent reports indicate that β3-ARs are also expressed in heart, blood vessels, gall bladder, gastrointestinal tract, prostate and urinary bladder detrusor, and brain [96, 97]. Concerning the role of β3-ARs in the retina, there are earlier observations indicating the existence of a relationship between β3-AR gene polymorphism and the development of proliferative diabetic retinopathy in patients with diabetes [98]. In addition, β3-AR activation has been reported to induce markers of angiogenesis in human retinal endothelial cells [44]. β3-ARs are localized to blood vessels in rodent retinas [47, 48] and they are up-regulated by hypoxia in OIR mice [48, 75]. In particular, β3-AR up-regulation in OIR C57BL/6J mice is particularly evident at the level of the growing endothelium of neovascular retinal tufts [48], suggesting a function of these receptors in the formation of this characteristic sign of aberrant neo-angiogenesis. Noteworthy, β3-AR up-regulation is unexpectedly strong in the retina of OIR 129S6 mice, where a more than ten-fold increase of β3-AR mRNA expression has been reported [75], and it is much higher than that observed in the retina of OIR C57BL/6 mice [48]. Thus, this dramatic increase in the expression of β3-ARs, which are only minimally blocked by propranolol [99], may be responsible, at least in part, for the strong aggressiveness of neovascularization in 129S6 mice and for the reported insensitivity to propranolol in this strain [75], as reported above. The demonstration that β3-ARs are involved in the regulation of the neovascular response in the retina comes from studies in mouse retinal explants, where β3-ARs have been found to modulate hypoxia-induced VEGF release. In particular, β3-AR activation with BRL37344, a selective β3-AR agonist, increases VEGF release, while β3-AR inhibition with SR59230A or L-748,337, two structurally different β3-AR blockers, or β3-AR silencing with specific siRNAs drastically down-regulate the hypoxic levels of VEGF [100]. In addition, studies with retinal explants also provide evidence for the involvement of the nitric oxide (NO) signaling pathway in mediating the β3-AR modulation of VEGF release. Indeed, there is evidence supporting NO as a downstream effector of β3-ARs in different cell types [101-103], and results in hypoxic retinal explants show that β3-AR activation increases VEGF release through the production of NO, while β3-AR blockade or β3-AR silencing have the opposite effects [100]. On the other hand, experiments investigating the effects of β3-AR blockade in the OIR C57BL/6J mouse model have shown that subcutaneous administration of SR59230A are devoid of effects, thus suggesting a minor role, if any, of β3-ARs in regulating retinal pathological angiogenesis [46]. Therefore, the observed potent effect of β3-AR blockade on VEGF release in retinal explants can be explained by assuming that, in OIR, systemic administration of SR59230A does not provide the retina with a sufficient drug concentration to interfere with VEGF release. In this respect, SR59230A at concentrations lower than 10 μM does not affect VEGF release in retinal explants [100].

Another possibility is that different post-receptor mechanisms may be activated in retinal explants and OIR. For instance, β3-ARs may hetero-oligomerize with β2-ARs, generating a β-adrenergic signaling unit with functional properties distinct from those of β2- and β3-ARs [104]. Since the formation of hetero-oligomers between membrane receptors is influenced by oxidative stress caused by hypoxia-ischemia [105-106], we cannot exclude that differences in oxygen tension in the two models (1% oxygen in retinal explants and atmospheric oxygen tension in OIR) may be responsible for the different outcomes of β3-AR blockade in retinal explants and in the OIR model.

Study in β1/β2 Knockout Mice

To get insights on the relative role of β2- and β3-ARs in the OIR model, a study has been performed in β1/2-AR knockout (KO) mice [107]. The results showed that, in the absence of β1- and β2-ARs, the NE up-regulation that characterizes OIR is decreased, suggesting that β1- and/or β2-ARs may contribute to regulate NE levels in the retina. In addition, the up-regulation of β3-ARs observed in the retina of OIR mice [48, 75] is not influenced by β1/2-AR deletion, excluding that the lack of β1- and/or β2-ARs may affect the expression of β3-ARs [107]. Retinal vascularization of KO mice maintained in normoxia is not significantly different from that of WT in terms of retinal coverage or morphology. In contrast, retinas of OIR KO mice are clearly different from those of WT. Indeed, as OIR retinas in WT are characterized by a pronounced avascular area and a number of neovascular tufts, similar to those observed in OIR C57BL/6J mice [26], the retinas of OIR KO mice display a significantly reduced avascular area and only a few neovascular tufts. These data show an impressive effect of β1/β2-AR deletion in OIR, and suggest that in OIR β-AR overstimulation may potentially act as a proangiogenic switch [107]. Although the effect of β1/2-AR deletion on retinal neovascularization are similar to those observed after β1/2-AR blockade [48, 73], at variance with β1/2-AR deletion, β1/2-AR blockade does not prevent the formation of the central avascular area presumably because the administration of β-AR blockers begins at PD12 when the avascular area is already formed [107]. Regarding angiogenic factors, OIR retinas of WT and KO mice show similar levels of VEGF, but differ in VEGF receptor (VEGFR) expression with VEGFR-1 in WT lower than in KO and VEGFR-2 in WT higher than in KO, consistent with a reduced angiogenic drive in KO retinas [107]. Indeed,

VEGF preferentially binds to VEGFR-1, which, according to its function as a decoy receptor [108], would reduce VEGFR-2 signaling thus interfering with the main role of VEGFR-2 in angiogenic processes [109]. However, the reduced VEGFR-2 signaling that characterizes KO is not sufficient to prevent BRB dysfunction, possibly because newly formed vessels colonizing the avascular area remain leaky until PD17 thus permitting the extravasation of plasma proteins or because VEGFR-2 signaling alone is not responsible for BRB leakage, which, instead, requires cross-communication between VEGFR-1 and VEGFR [107].

Interestingly, in KO mice selective β3-AR activation may replace β2-AR function. Indeed, in OIR KO mice the administration of BRL37344 leads to a formation of retinal neovascular tufts that are similar to that observed in the retina of BRL37344-treated OIR WT [107]. In this respect, one can assume that β2-ARs may normally mask β3-AR activity suggesting a redundancy of the β-AR system. The finding that β3-AR activation sustains the angiogenic response in the absence of β1- and β2-ARs may help to explain the discrepancy between our studies reporting anti-angiogenic effects of propranolol in C57BL/6J mice [48, 73] and those excluding propranolol effects in 129S6 mice, where the OIR model is characterized by an enormous increase of β3-AR expression [75].

Overall, the results from our studies confirm the pivotal role that β2-ARs play in retinal angiogenesis thus expanding the importance of the use of β-AR blockers to counteract angiogenesis-driven retinal pathologies. As to β3-ARs, the fact that their agonism increases the neovascular response in WT and causes neovascularization in KO mice indicates that, in the presence of β1- and/or β2-ARs, β3-ARs may potentiate the retinal angiogenic responses, whereas, in their absence, β3-ARs may sustain the angiogenic drive.

The studies in animal models have provided a considerable amount of data indicating that, at least in OIR C57BL/6J mice, β-AR blockade, and in particular β2-AR blockade, may play a significant action against hypoxia-induced retinal neovascularization. This evidence has prompted an interest in exploring the possibility that the administration of a β2-AR or a β1/β2-AR antagonist, such as propranolol, may help in the treatment of ROP [110-112].

From Bench to Bedside: Clinical Trials Evaluating Propranolol Treatment in Preterm Newborns with ROP

To verify whether propranolol could be useful in reducing the progression of ROP, a first randomized controlled pilot clinical trial was performed to evaluate safety and efficacy of oral propranolol administration in preterm newborns affected by an advanced phase of ROP [110, 112].

In that study, a total of 52 preterm newborns with gestational age < 32 weeks and stage 2 ROP without plus in zone II were enrolled. Treated and control newborns with a 1:1 allocation in blocks of 8 were randomized and stratified in 2 groups with gestational age of 23-25 and of 26-32 weeks; they were alternated between propranolol added to standard treatment or standard treatment alone (the treatment adopted by the Early Treatment of Retinopathy of Prematurity Cooperative Group) [6]. Exclusion criteria included newborns with congenital or acquired cardiovascular anomalies, renal failure or cerebral hemorrhage at enrollment, and newborns with ROP in zone I or at a more advanced stage than stage 2 without plus in zone II. With severe adverse effects related to propranolol (severe bradycardia, hypotension, or wheezing), the administration of propranolol was permanently discontinued. Treated newborns were randomized at 67 ± 14 days postnatal age (weight 1678 ± 393 g), while control newborns were randomized at 68 ± 17 days postnatal age (weight 1559 ± 431 g). The first 4 newborns in the treated group with gestational age of 23-25 weeks (n = 12) and all the newborns in the treated group with gestational age of 26-32 weeks (n = 14) were treated with 0.5 mg/kg/6 hours propranolol (high-dose). After the appearance of severe adverse events in 3 newborns in the 23-25 weeks group, the dosage was reduced, and the remaining 8 newborns were treated with 0.25 mg/kg/6 hours (low-dose). Newborns received propranolol for an average of 66.1 ± 31 days (range, 6-90 days): 60.2 ± 35 days (range, 6-90 days) in the 23-25 weeks group, 71.2 ± 28 days (range, 8-90 days) in the 26-32 weeks group. All the newborns with gestational age < 32 weeks had ophthalmologic evaluations through indirect ophthalmoscopy [113]. When ROP in zone II reached stage 2 without plus, newborns were enrolled, and ophthalmologic examinations were scheduled weekly or more frequently, according to the severity of ROP. Propranolol was administered orally as 2 mg/ml syrup shortly after feeding. The treatment was continued until complete development of retinal vascularization, although administration was not permitted for more than 90 days. The physicians and nurses were aware of the allocated arm, but the ophthalmologists and data analysts were blinded to the allocation. When ROP reached stage 2 or 3 with plus disease, the newborns were treated with peripheral retinal ablation performed by conventional laser photocoagulation [6]. An intravitreal bevacizumab injection was considered as rescue treatment for more aggressive ROP with insufficient regression after laser treatment [114]. Vitrectomy was considered in newborns with ROP stage 4A to reduce tractional retinal detachment from fibrous proliferation. Vital signs and respiratory and hemodynamic variables were monitored continuously. Blood gas analysis, glucose, serum electrolyte levels, liver and renal function tests, complete blood cell count, and C-reactive protein level were measured once a week for the first 3 weeks after randomization. Standard electrocardiogram and cardiac ultrasounds were performed weekly for 3 weeks. Plasma propranolol was measured on dried blood spots by a liquid-chromatography tandem-mass spectrometry method [115] during the first 3 days of treatment and at the steady state on the 10th day of treatment [116]. Plasma levels of VEGF and of soluble E-selectin (sE-selectin), a soluble cell adhesion molecule regarded as a biomarker of inflammatory processes whose plasma levels are closely correlated to ROP [117], were also evaluated.

The primary indicator of the efficacy of the propranolol treatment in reducing the progression of ROP was the different incidence of the progression of the disease from stage 2 ROP without plus to stage 2 ROP with plus and to stage 3 with or without plus between treated and control groups. Newborns treated with propranolol showed less progression to stage 3 (risk ratio 0.52; 95% confidence interval 0.47-0.58; relative reduction of risk 48%) or stage 3 plus (relative risk 0.42; 95% confidence interval 0.31-0.58; relative reduction of risk 58%). Other indicators included the different incidence of the treatment with laser photocoagulation, the rescue treatment with bevacizumab, the progression to stage 4 or 5 ROP, and the different need for vitrectomy. The results of this study demonstrated a reduced need for laser photocoagulation treatment in newborns receiving propranolol. The number of newborns and eyes treated with bevacizumab was lower in the treated group than in the control group (relative risk 0.48; 95% confidential interval 0.29-0.79; relative reduction of risk 52%), and no newborns progressed to stage 4. In the majority of treated newborns after 10-15 days of treatment, the ridge tended to turn pale and a second, more peripheral ridge appeared usually on 2 or 3 quadrants. After 1 month, the peripheral ridge was more evident than the first one, which disappeared after 2 months of therapy, leaving just a thin demarcation line. After approximately 2 months, the normal retinal vessels also passed over the peripheral ridge, which was reduced in width and height. Overall, these results demonstrated that propranolol is effective in counteracting ROP progression and promotes normal vessel growth into the avascular zone of the retina, thus reducing the impact of the disease. In addition, plasma levels of sE-selectin were reduced in propranolol-treated newborns starting from 7 days of treatment, while the drug did not affect plasma levels of VEGF. The reduced level of sE-selectin is another sign of the anti-angiogenic effect of propranolol as sE-selectin is involved in angiogenesis and capillary morphogenesis and its plasma levels are related to ROP [117]. The fact that the plasma levels of VEGF were not affected by propranolol, regardless to the administered dose, is of particular importance for the risk concerns relative to the systemic administration of propranolol. Indeed, as demonstrated in mouse studies, VEGF participates in brain morphogenesis and severe reductions of VEGF result in degeneration of the cerebral cortex [118, 119].

However, despite the effectiveness of propranolol in preventing ROP progression, this study suggested that systemic administration of propranolol is not sufficiently safe. Indeed, premature newborns with ROP have a high risk of associated complications that could make propranolol unsafe, although this drug is generally well tolerated in newborns and infants and has been used for decades in term newborns for cardiovascular indications [116]. Overall, during the 90 days of the study, the hemodynamic and respiratory variables did not differ between the treated and the control groups. Weight gain was comparable in both groups. During the first 3 weeks of the study, the variables of blood gas analysis, blood glucose, serum sodium and chloride, liver and renal function tests, complete blood cell count, and C-reactive protein levels were comparable in the 2 groups. Only potassium values were significantly greater in the treated group, although all values were within the normal range. In addition, no differences were observed in the laboratory tests as well as in respiratory and hemodynamic variables between newborns of gestational age of 23-25 weeks treated with high-dose or with low-dose propranolol. No newborns required treatment with inotropes during the study period. No newborns in either group had electrocardiographic and/or cardiac ultrasound abnormalities. A series of apneas, bradycardias, and hypotension were observed in 3 newborns in the group with gestational age of 23-25 weeks treated with high-dose propranolol. Two newborns with gestational age of 24^{+6} weeks developed these symptoms simultaneously with the development of an infection. Another newborn with gestational age of 24^{+5} weeks on the 36th day of treatment had these findings, in conjunction with the induction of general anesthesia before neurosurgery. All these newborns were resuscitated: one recovered with the administration of adrenaline, and the others, who were refractory to adrenaline, recovered after receiving terlipressin. The protocol was amended, and one-half dose was then used for newborns in the group with gestational age of 23-25 weeks. However, another newborn with gestational age of 23^{+2} weeks on the 6th day of treatment had severe apneas and bradycardia after respiratory failure attributable to massive atelectasis; this newborn responded to the administration of adrenaline. Severe bradycardia occurred after 28 days of treatment in one newborn with gestational age of 30 weeks simultaneously with the development of an H1N1 virus infection. Another newborn with gestational age of 26^{+4} weeks had severe bronchospasm after 8 days of treatment but responded to the administration of adrenaline.

Overall, this trial demonstrated that, in stable preterm newborns, treatment with propranolol is definitely well tolerated, as demonstrated by the stability of the biochemical, hematologic, hemodynamic, and respiratory variables. But, when propranolol was administered to unstable preterm newborns, there was a high risk of hypotension and bradycardia that are sometimes unresponsive to catecholamines. In contrast to infants and children, in whom adverse events after treatment with propranolol are usually mild and not life-threatening, preterm newborns appear to have a greater risk of developing severe adverse effects when complications frequently associated with prematurity, like sepsis, develop during treatment with β-blockers. Because of the increased stiffness of their myocardium, neonates possess a limited ability to increase their cardiac output by increasing stroke volume, and their cardiac output is significantly dependent on heart rate [120]. Because myocardial depression is a well-known manifestation of organ dysfunction in sepsis, treatment with β-blockers may prevent the only compensatory mechanism to increase the myocardial function.

Limitations of this study may be found in the fact that it was planned as a pilot study with a small number of enrolled patients. In addition, the study was not placebo-controlled, and only the ophthalmologists were blinded. This strategy was chosen to identify any possible adverse effects and immediately discontinue the administration of propranolol. Many uncertainties still remain. First, propranolol was chosen in doses that usually do not produce adverse effects but are effective in the treatment of infantile hemangiomas [38]. However, it is unknown at what concentration, when administered orally, propranolol reaches the retina. Second, it was not possible to estimate the optimal start and duration of administration.

A second randomized controlled pilot clinical trial performed to evaluate safety and efficacy of oral propranolol [111] gave similar results. In this study, twenty preterm newborns with gestational age of 24-28 weeks and birth weight < 1500 g were randomized either to oral propranolol (n = 10) or placebo (n = 10). They had evidence for ROP with any of the following: stage 1 (zone I); stage 2 or higher (zones I or II); and/or plus disease. Propranolol safety, ROP progression and need for invasive intervention were evaluated. Propranolol was given for 4 weeks or until ROP resolution or hospital discharge. During treatment, vital signs and blood glucose levels, platelet counts, ECG and echocardiography were checked. Propranolol was started with a dose of 0.16 mg/kg body weight every 8h. Placebo was given in similar volume to that of propranolol. In the absence of side effects, the dose was incrementally increased daily to a maximum of 0.67 mg/kg every 8h. Newborns of the placebo group required twice as many interventions as those treated with propranolol. Indeed, in the propranolol group 21% of the treated eyes required laser intervention compared to 42% in the placebo group. However, this result was not statistically significant, possibly because the small sample size. At variance of the study of Filippi et al. [110], the study of Makhoul et al. [111] showed instead that none of the known side effects of propranolol occurred in treated newborns, suggesting that systemic propranolol is safe in preterm newborns.

In conclusion, two pilot clinical trials [110, 111] suggest that treatment with propranolol is effective in counteracting the progression of ROP and add new perspectives for the treatment of this and other proliferative retinopathies. Nevertheless, the high incidence of adverse effects highlighted in the study of Filippi et al. [110] suggests that systemic administration is not sufficiently safe. A future objective will be to explore and develop topical delivery systems to ensure high retinal and low plasma concentrations of propranolol.

In this regard, a new clinical study with propranolol eye drops administered to newborns with ROP stage 2 zone II without plus has been recently performed by Filippi et al. (data still unpublished). The objective of this study was to demonstrate that propranolol treatment is able to reduce the percentage of progression of ROP to stage 2 or 3 with plus disease at less than 18% (the percentage observed after oral propranolol treatment). After the diagnosis of stage 2 without plus, newborns were treated with 3 micro drops of 0.1% propranolol in each eye, three times a day, for a maximum period of 90 days or until the complete vascularization of the retina. Unfortunately, the number of newborns in which ROP progressed to stage 2 or 3 with plus disease was around 25%. Even though the objective was not reached, the results were substantially similar to those obtained after oral administration of propranolol, but no adverse effect were observed, and propranolol plasma levels were significantly lower than those measured after oral administration. In conclusion, this study suggests that topical administration of propranolol could be an effective strategy to counteract ROP progression. A new trial is now ongoing, were propranolol eye drops are administered to preterm newborns at a higher concentration and in a more precocious stage (ROP stage 1) to ensure a longer period of exposition to propranolol.

Conclusion

ROP remains an elusive disease. The application of ETROP criteria (ablation of the non-vascularized retina) can reduce blindness, but many treated patients have a poor outcome. Our studies in a mouse model of ROP have demonstrated that retinal NE increases in response to hypoxia and β-ARs may regulate VEGF production and retinal neovascularization. Noteworthy, these studies have shown that significant reduction of neovascularization can be achieved by β-AR blockade, suggesting the possible therapeutic use of β-AR blockers to counteract retinal neovascularization in ROP. The pilot study with oral propranolol on the one hand has established the efficacy of propranolol treatment, while on the other has indicated that the safety is a concern.

To overcome these safety problems, a more appropriate way of propranolol delivery is needed, such as topical propranolol application. Results obtained in an ongoing clinical trial with propranolol eye drops are expected to help the development of safe propranolol treatments for ROP. Whether the concerns about propranolol safety will be overcome, thus propranolol could be regarded as a promising new therapeutic tool for the treatment of ROP. Similar experimentations might be extended to other proliferative retinal diseases for which oral treatment with propranolol is currently under investigation, such as choroidal hemangioma in Sturge-Weber disease, periocular hemangiomas, diabetic retinopathy, and AMD [70, 121-123].

Acknowledgments

The authors thank Prof. Giovanni Casini for critical reading of the manuscript. Special thanks are due to our mentor, Prof. Paola Bagnoli, whose contribution to these studies has been fundamental.

References

[1] Palmer, E. A., Hardy, R. J., Dobson, V., Phelps, D. L., Quinn, G. E., Summers, C. G., Krom, C. P., Tung, B. Cryotherapy for Retinopathy of Prematurity Cooperative Group. 15-year outcomes following threshold retinopathy of prematurity: final results from the multicenter trial of cryotherapy for retinopathy of prematurity. *Arch Ophthalmol,* 2005, 123, 311-318.

[2] Cryotherapy for Retinopathy of Prematurity Cooperative Group. Multicenter trial of cryotherapy for retinopathy of prematurity-preliminary results. *Arch Ophthalmol,* 1988, 106, 471-479.

[3] Cryotherapy for Retinopathy of Prematurity Cooperative Group. Multicenter trial of cryotherapy for retinopathy of prematurity: ophthalmological outcomes at 10 years. *Arch Ophthalmol,* 2001, 119, 1110-1118.

[4] Connolly, B. P., Ng, E. Y., McNamara, J. A., Regillo, C. D., Vander, J. F., Tasman, W. A comparison of laser photocoagulation with cryotherapy for threshold retinopathy of prematurity at 10 years: part 2. Refractive outcome. *Ophthalmology,* 2002, 109, 936-941.

[5] Ng, E. Y., Connolly, B. P., McNamara, J. A., Regillo, C. D., Vander, J. F., Tasman, W. A comparison of laser photocoagulation with cryotherapy for threshold retinopathy of prematurity at 10 years: part 1. Visual function and structural outcome. *Ophthalmology,* 2002, 109, 928-934.

[6] Early Treatment for Retinopathy of Prematurity Cooperative Group. Revised indications for treatment of retinopathy of prematurity: results of the Early Treatment for Retinopathy of Prematurity Randomized Trial. *Arch Ophthalmol,* 2003, 121, 1684-1696.

[7] An International Committee for the Classification of Retinopathy of Prematurity. The International Classification of Retinopathy of Prematurity revisited. *Arch Ophthalmol,* 2005,123, 991-999.

[8] Fleck, B. W. Management of retinopathy of prematurity. *Arch Dis Child Fetal Neonatal Ed*, 2013, 98, F454-F456.

[9] Tokunaga, C. C., Mitton, K. P., Dailey, W., Massoll, C., Roumayah, K., Tarabishy, N., Cheng, M., Guzman, E., Drenser, K. A. Effect of anti-VEGF treatment on developing retina following oxygen-induced retinopathy. *Invest Ophthalmol Vis Sci,* 2014, 55, 1884-1892.

[10] Chowers, I., Banin, E., Hemo, Y., Porat, R., Falk, H., Keshet, E., Pe'er, J., Panet, A. Gene transfer by viral vectors into blood vessels in a rat model of retinopathy of prematurity. *Br J Ophthalmol,* 2001, 85, 991-995.

[11] Rajappa, M., Saxena, P., Kaur, J. Ocular angiogenesis: mechanisms and recent advances in therapy. *Adv Clin Chem,* 2010, 50, 103-121.

[12] Connor, K. M., San Giovanni, J. P., Lofqvist, C., Aderman, C. M., Chen, J., Higuchi, A., Hong, S., Pravda, E. A., Majchrzak, S., Carper, D., Hellstrom, A., Kang, J. X., Chew, E. Y., Salem, N. Jr., Serhan, C. N., Smith, L. E. Increased dietary intake of omega-3-polyunsaturated fatty acids reduces pathological retinal angiogenesis. *Nat Med,* 2007, 13, 868-873.

[13] Stahl, A., Sapieha, P., Connor, K. M., Sangiovanni, J. P., Chen, J., Aderman, C. M., Willett, K. L., Krah, N. M., Dennison, R. J., Seaward, M. R., Guerin, K., Hua, J., Smith L. E. Short communication: PPAR gamma mediates a direct antiangiogenic effect of omega 3-PUFAs in proliferative retinopathy. *Circ Res,* 2010, 107, 495-500.

[14] Löfqvist, C., Niklasson, A., Engström, E., Friberg, L. E., Camacho-Hübner, C., Ley, D., Borg, J., Smith, L. E., Hellström, A. A pharmacokinetic and dosing study of intravenous insulin-like growth factor-I and IGF-binding protein-3 complex to preterm infants. *Pediatr Res,* 2009, 65, 574-579.

[15] Smith, L. E. Pathogenesis of retinopathy of prematurity. *Acta Paediatr Suppl,* 2002, 91, 26-28.

[16] Grossniklaus, H. E., Kang, S. J., Berglin, L. Animal models of choroidal and retinal neovascularization. *Prog Retin Eye Res,* 2010, 29, 500-519.

[17] Heidary, G., Vanderveen, D., Smith, L. E. Retinopathy of prematurity: current concepts in molecular pathogenesis. *Semin Ophthalmol,* 2009, 24, 77-81.

[18] Chen, J., Smith, L. E. Retinopathy of prematurity. *Angiogenesis,* 2007, 10, 133-140.

[19] Ashton, N., Ward, B., Serpell, G. Effect of oxygen on developing retinal vessels with particular reference to the problem of retrolental fibroplasia. *Br J Ophthalmol,* 1954, 38, 397-432.

[20] Penn, J. S., Tolman, B. L., Lowery, L. A. Variable oxygen exposure causes preretinal neovascularization in the newborn rat. *Invest Ophthalmol Vis Sci,* 1993, 34, 576-585.

[21] Smith, L. E., Wesolowski, E., McLellan, A., Kostyk, S. K., D'Amato, R., Sullivan, R., D'Amato, P. A. Oxygen-induced retinopathy in the mouse. *Invest Ophthalmol Vis Sci,* 1994, 35, 101-111.

[22] McLeod, D. S., Brownstein, R., Lutty, G. A. Vaso-obliteration in the canine model of oxygen-induced retinopathy. *Invest Ophthalmol Vis Sci,* 1996, 37, 300-311.

[23] Cao, R., Jensen, L., Söll, I., Hauptmann, G., Cao, Y. Hypoxia-induced retinal angiogenesis in zebrafish as a model to study retinopathy. *PLoS ONE,* 2008, 3, e2748.

[24] McLeod, D. S., D'Anna, S. A., Lutty, G. A. Clinical and histopathologic features of canine oxygen-induced proliferative retinopathy. *Invest Ophthalmol Vis Sci,* 1998, 39, 1918-1932.

[25] Madan, A., Penn, J. S. Animal models of oxygen-induced retinopathy. *Front Biosci,* 2003, 8, d1030-d1043.

[26] Stahl, A., Connor, K. M., Sapieha, P., Chen, J., Dennison, R. J., Krah, N. M., Seaward, M. R., Willett, K. L., Aderman, C. M., Guerin, K. I., Hua, J., Löfqvist, C., Hellström, A., Smith, L. E. The mouse retina as an angiogenesis model. *Invest Ophthalmol Vis Sci,* 2010, 51, 2813-2826.

[27] Aguilar, E., Dorrell, M. I., Friedlander, D., Jacobson, R. A., Johnson, A., Marchetti, V., Moreno, S. K., Ritter, M. R., Friedlander, M. Ocular models of angiogenesis. *Methods Enzymol,* 2008, 444, 115-158.

[28] Lange, C., Ehlken, C., Stahl, A., Martin, G., Hansen, L., Agostini, H. T. Kinetics of retinal vaso-obliteration and neovascularisation in the oxygen-induced retinopathy (OIR) mouse model. *Graefes Arch Clin Exp Ophthalmol,* 2009, 247, 1205-1211.

[29] Gu, X., Samuel, S., El-Shabrawey, M., Caldwell, R. B., Bartoli, M., Marcus, D. M., Brooks, S. E. Effects of sustained hyperoxia on revascularization in experimental retinopathy of prematurity. *Invest Ophthalmol Vis Sci,* 2002, 43, 496-502.

[30] Ozaki, H., Yu, A. Y., Della, N., Ozaki, K., Luna, J. D., Yamada, H., Hackett, S. F., Okamoto, N., Zack, D. J., Semenza, G. L., Campochiaro, P. A. Hypoxia inducible factor-1alpha is increased in ischemic retina: temporal and spatial correlation with VEGF expression. Invest *Ophthalmol Vis Sci,* 1999, 40, 182-189.

[31] Smith, L. E., Shen, W., Perruzzi, C., Soker, S., Kinose, F., Xu, X., Robinson, G., Driver, S., Bischoff, J., Zhang, B., Schaeffer, J. M., Senger, D. R. Regulation of vascular endothelial growth factor-dependent retinal neovascularization by insulin-like growth factor-1 receptor. *Nat Med,* 1999, 5, 1390-1395.

[32] Davies, M. H., Stempel, A. J., Powers, M. R. MCP-1 deficiency delays regression of pathologic retinal neovascularization in a model of ischemic retinopathy. *Invest Ophthalmol Vis Sci,* 2008, 49, 4195-4202.

[33] Chan, C. K., Pham, L. N., Zhou, J., Spee, C., Ryan, S. J., Hinton, D. R. Differential expression of pro- and antiangiogenic factors in mouse strain-dependent hypoxia-induced retinal neovascularization. *Lab Invest,* 2005, 85, 721-733.

[34] Ritter, M. R., Banin, E., Moreno, S. K., Aguilar, E., Dorrell, M. I., Friedlander, M. Myeloid progenitors differentiate into microglia and promote vascular repair in a model of ischemic retinopathy. *J Clin Invest,* 2006, 116, 3266-3276.

[35] Hemangioma Investigator Group, Haggstrom, A. N., Drolet, B. A., Baselga, E., Chamlin, S. L., Garzon, M. C., Horii, K. A., Lucky, A. W., Mancini, A. J., Metry, D. W., Newell, B., Nopper, A. J., Frieden, I. J. Prospective study of infantile hemangiomas: Demographic, prenatal, and perinatal characteristics. *J Pediatr,* 2007, 150, 291-294.

[36] Kleinman, M. E., Greives, M. R., Churgin, S. S., Blechman, K. M., Chang, E. I., Ceradini, D. J., Tepper, O. M., Gurtner, G. C. Hypoxia-induced mediators of stem/progenitor cell trafficking are increased in children with hemangioma. *Arterioscler Thromb Vasc Biol,* 2007, 27, 2664-2670.

[37] Przewratil, P., Sitkiewicz, A., Andrzejewska, E. Local serum levels of vascular endothelial growth factor in infantile hemangioma: intriguing mechanism of endothelial growth. *Cytokine,* 2010, 49, 141-147.

[38] Léauté-Labrèze, C., Dumas de la Roque, E., Hubiche, T., Boralevi, F., Thambo, J. B., Taieb, A. Propranolol for severe hemangiomas of infancy. *N Engl J Med,* 2008, 358, 2649-2651.

[39] Sans, V., de la Roque, E. D., Berge, J., Grenier, N., Boralevi, F., Mazereeuw-Hautier, J., Lipsker, D., Dupuis, E., Ezzedine, K., Vergnes, P., Taieb, A., Léauté-Labrèze, C. Propranolol for severe infantile hemangiomas: Follow-up report. *Pediatrics,* 2009, 124, e423-e431.

[40] Ji, Y., Chen, S., Li, K., Li, L., Xu, C., Xiang, B. Signaling pathways in the development of infantile hemangioma. *J Hematol Oncol,* 2014, 7,13.

[41] Chim, H., Armijo, B. S., Miller, E., Gliniak, C., Serret, M. A., Gosain, A. K. Propranolol induces regression of hemangioma cells through HIF-1alpha-mediated inhibition of VEGF-A. *Ann Surg,* 2012, 256, 146-156.

[42] Casini, G., Dal Monte, M., Fornaciari, I., Filippi, L., Bagnoli, P. The β-adrenergic system as a possible new target for pharmacologic treatment of neovascular retinal diseases. *Prog Retin Eye Res,* 2014, 42, 103-129.

[43] Walker, R. J., Steinle, J. J. Role of beta-adrenergic receptors in inflammatory marker expression in Muller cells. *Invest Ophthalmol Vis Sci,* 2007, 48, 5276-5281.

[44] Steinle, J. J., Booz, G. W., Meininger, C. J., Day, J. N., Granger, H. J. Beta 3-adrenergic receptors regulate retinal endothelial cell migration and proliferation. *J Biol Chem,* 2003, 278, 20681-20686.

[45] Ferrari-Dileo, G. Beta 1 and beta 2 adrenergic binding sites in bovine retina and retinal blood vessels. *Invest Ophthalmol Vis Sci,* 1988, 29, 695-699.

[46] Martini, D., Dal Monte, M., Ristori, C., Cupisti, E., Mei, S., Fiorini, P., Filippi, L., Bagnoli, P. Antiangiogenic effects of beta2 -adrenergic receptor blockade in a mouse model of oxygen-induced retinopathy. *J Neurochem,* 2011, 119, 1317-1329.

[47] Mori, A., Miwa, T., Sakamoto, K., Nakahara, T., Ishii, K. Pharmacological evidence for the presence of functional beta(3)-adrenoceptors in rat retinal blood vessels. *Naunyn Schmiedebergs Arch Pharmacol,* 2010, 382, 119-126.

[48] Ristori, C., Filippi, L., Dal Monte, M., Martini, D., Cammalleri, M., Fortunato, P., la Marca, G., Fiorini, P., Bagnoli, P. Role of the adrenergic system in a mouse model of oxygen-induced retinopathy: antiangiogenic effects of beta-adrenoreceptor blockade. *Invest Ophthalmol Vis Sci,* 2011, 52, 155-170.

[49] Hadjiconstantinou, M., Cohen, J., Neff, N. H. Epinephrine: a potential neurotransmitter in retina. *J Neurochem,* 1983, 41, 1440-1444.

[50] Delaey, C., van De Voorde, J. Regulatory mechanisms in the retinal and choroidal circulation. *Ophthalmic Res,* 2000, 32, 249-256.

[51] Osborne, N. N., Patel, S. The presence of dopamine-β-hydroxylase-like enzyme in the vertebrate retina. *Neurochem Int,* 1985, 7, 51-56.

[52] Fukuda, M., Ishimoto, I., Kuwayama, Y., Shimizu, Y., Shiosaka, S., Takagi, H., Tohyama, M. Monoamine accumulating neuron system in the rat retina with special reference to noradrenaline accumulating neurons. *Exp Eye Res,* 1982, 34, 487-491.

[53] Osborne, N. N. Noradrenaline, a transmitter candidate in the retina. *J Neurochem,* 1981, 36, 17-27.

[54] Chen, Z., Jia, W., Kaufman, P. L., Cynader, M. Immunohistochemical localization of dopamine-beta-hydroxylase in human and monkey eyes. *Curr Eye Res,* 1999, 18, 39-48.

[55] Sorriento, D., Santulli, G., Del Giudice, C., Anastasio, A., Trimarco, B., Iaccarino, G. Endothelial cells are able to synthesize and release

catecholamines both *in vitro* and *in vivo*. *Hypertension,* 2012, 60, 129-136.

[56] Dal Monte, M., Martini, D., Latina, V., Pavan, B., Filippi, L., Bagnoli, P. Beta-adrenoreceptor agonism influences retinal responses to hypoxia in a model of retinopathy of prematurity. *Invest Ophthalmol Vis Sci,* 2012, 53, 2181-2192.

[57] Ray, K., Dutta, A., Panjwani, U., Thakur, L., Anand, J. P., Kumar, S. Hypobaric hypoxia modulates brain biogenic amines and disturbs sleep architecture. *Neurochem Int,* 2011, 58, 112-118.

[58] Chen, X. Q., Du, J. Z., Wang, Y. S. Regulation of hypoxia-induced release of corticotropin-releasing factor in the rat hypothalamus by norepinephrine. *Regul Pept,* 2004, 119, 221-228.

[59] Jiang,Y., Walker, R. J., Kern, T. S., Steinle, J. J. Application of isoproterenol inhibits diabetic-like changes in the rat retina. *Exp Eye Res,* 2010, 91, 171-179.

[60] Steinle, J. J., Kern, T. S., Thomas, S. A., McFadyen-Ketchum, L. S., Smith,C. P. Increased basement membrane thickness, pericyte ghosts, and loss of retinal thickness and cells in dopamine beta hydroxylase knockout mice. *Exp Eye Res,* 2009, 88, 1014-1019.

[61] Wiley, L. A., Rupp, G. R., Steinle, J. J. Sympathetic innervation regulates basement membrane thickening and pericyte number in rat retina. *Invest Ophthalmol Vis Sci,* 2005, 46, 744-748.

[62] Kaur, C., Foulds, W. S., Ling, E. A. Blood-retinal barrier in hypoxic ischaemic conditions: basic concepts, clinical features and management. *Prog Retin Eye Res,* 2008, 27, 622-647.

[63] Poulaki, V., Joussen, A. M., Mitsiades, N., Mitsiades, C. S., Iliaki, E. F., Adamis, A. P. Insulin-like growth factor-I plays a pathogenetic role in diabetic retinopathy. *Am J Pathol,* 2004, 165, 457-469.

[64] Smith, L. E. IGF-1 and retinopathy of prematurity in the preterm infant. *Biol Neonate,* 2005, 88, 237-244.

[65] Shyu, K. G., Liou, J. Y., Wang, B. W., Fang, W. J., Chang, H. Carvedilol prevents cardiac hypertrophy and overexpression of hypoxia-inducible factor-1alpha and vascular endothelial growth factor in pressure-overloaded rat heart. *J Biomed Sci,* 2005, 12, 409-420.

[66] Bartoli, M., Al-Shabrawey, M., Labazi, M., Behzadian, M. A., Istanboli, M., El-Remessy, A. B., Caldwell, R. W., Marcus, D. M., Caldwell, R. B. HMG-CoA reductase inhibitors (statin) prevents retinal neovascularization in a model of oxygen-induced retinopathy. *Invest Ophthalmol Vis Sci,* 2009, 50, 4934-4940.

[67] Ricci, B., Ricci, F., Maggiano, N. Oxygen-induced retinopathy in the newborn rat: morphological and immunohistological findings in animals treated with topical timolol maleate. *Ophthalmologica,* 2000, 214, 136-139.

[68] Ricci, B., Minicucci, G., Manfredi, A., Santo, A. Oxygen-induced retinopathy in the newborn rat: effects of hyperbarism and topical administration of timolol maleate. *Graefes Arch Clin Exp Ophthalmol,* 1995, 233, 226-230.

[69] Ricci, B., Calogero, G., Caprilli, A., Quaranta-Leoni, F. M. Reduced severity of oxygen-induced retinopathy in the newborn rat after topical administration of timolol maleate. A preliminary study. *Doc Ophthalmol,* 1991, 77, 47-56.

[70] Montero, J. A., Ruiz-Moreno, J. M., Sanchis-Merino, E., Perez-Martin, S. Systemic beta-blockers may reduce the need for repeated intravitreal injections in patients with wet age-related macular degeneration treated by bevacizumab. *Retina,* 2013, 33, 508-512.

[71] Lavine, J. A., Sang, Y., Wang, S., Ip, M. S., Sheibani, N. Attenuation of choroidal neovascularization by beta(2)-adrenoreceptor antagonism. *JAMA Ophthalmol,* 2013, 131, 376-382.

[72] Schiestl, C., Neuhaus, K., Zoller, S., Subotic, U., Forster-Kuebler, I., Michels, R., Balmer, C., Weibel, L. Efficacy and safety of propranolol as first-line treatment for infantile hemangiomas. *Eur J Pediatr,* 2011, 170, 493-501.

[73] Dal Monte, M., Casini, G., la Marca, G., Isacchi, B., Filippi, L., Bagnoli, P. Eye drop propranolol administration promotes the recovery of oxygen-induced retinopathy in mice. *Exp Eye Res,* 2013, 111, 27-35.

[74] Padrini, L., Isacchi, B., Bilia, A. R., Pini, A., Lanzi, C., Masini, E., Della Bona, M. L., Calvani, A. M., Ceccantini, R., la Marca, G., Filippi, L. Pharmacokinetics and local safety profile of propranolol eye drops in rabbits. *Pediatr Res,* 2014, 76, 378-385.

[75] Chen, J., Joyal, J. S., Hatton, C. J., Juan, A. M., Pei, D. T., Hurst, C. G., Xu, D., Stahl, A., Hellström, A., Smith, L. E. Propranolol inhibition of beta-adrenergic receptor does not suppress pathologic neovascularization in oxygen-induced retinopathy. *Invest Ophthalmol Vis Sci,* 2012, 53, 2968-2977.

[76] Filippi, L., Dal Monte, M., Bagnoli, P. Different efficacy of propranolol in mice with oxygen-induced retinopathy: could differential effects of propranolol be related to differences in mouse strains? *Invest Ophthalmol Vis Sci,* 2012, 53, 7421-7423.

[77] Chen, J., Hellström, A., Smith, L. E. Author response: different efficacy of propranolol in mice with oxygen-induced retinopathy: could differential effects of propranolol be related to differences in mouse strains? *Invest Ophthalmol Vis Sci,* 2012, 53, 7728-7729.

[78] Good, W. V., Hardy, R. J., Dobson, V., Palmer, E. A., Phelps, D. L., Quintos, M., Tung, B., Early Treatment for Retinopathy of Prematurity Cooperative Group. The incidence and course of retinopathy of prematurity: findings from the early treatment for retinopathy of prematurity study. *Pediatrics,* 2005, 116, 15-23.

[79] Good, W. V., Hardy, R. J., Wallace, D. K., Bremer, D., Rogers, D. L., Siatkowski, R. M., de Becker, I., Summers, C. G., Fellows, R., Tung, B., Palmer, E. A. β-Blocking and racial variation in the severity of retinopathy of prematurity. *Arch Ophthalmol,* 2012, 130, 117-118.

[80] McLean, R. C., Baird, S. W., Becker, L. C., Townsend, S. N., Gerstenblith, G., Kass, D. A., Tomaselli, G. F., Schulman, S. P. Response to catecholamine stimulation of polymorphisms of the beta-1 and beta-2 adrenergic receptors. *Am J Cardiol,* 2012, 110, 1001-1007.

[81] Pierce, E. A., Avery, R. L., Foley, E. D., Aiello, L. P., Smith, L. E. Vascular endothelial growth factor/vascular permeability factor expression in a mouse model of retinal neovascularization. *Proc Natl Acad Sci USA,* 1995, 92, 905-909.

[82] Vrydag, W., Michel, M. C. Tools to study beta3-adrenoceptors. *Naunyn Schmiedebergs Arch Pharmacol,* 2007, 374, 385-398.

[83] Phipps, J. A., Wilkinson-Berka, J. L., Fletcher, E. L. Retinal dysfunction in diabetic ren-2 rats is ameliorated by treatment with valsartan but not atenolol. *Invest Ophthalmol Vis Sci,* 2007, 48, 927-934.

[84] Wilkinson-Berka, J. L., Tan, G., Jaworski, K., Ninkovic, S. Valsartan but not atenolol improves vascular pathology in diabetic Ren-2 rat retina. *Am J Hypertens,* 2007, 20, 423-430.

[85] Gagnon, A. W., Kallal, L., Benovic, J. L. Role of clathrin-mediated endocytosis in agonist-induced down-regulation of the beta2-adrenergic receptor. *J Biol Chem,* 1998, 273, 6976-6981.

[86] Nishikawa, M., Mak, J. C., Shirasaki, H., Barnes, P. J. Differential down-regulation of pulmonary beta 1- and beta 2-adrenoceptor messenger RNA with prolonged *in vivo* infusion of isoprenaline. *Eur J Pharmacol,* 1993, 247, 131-138.

[87] Gambarana, C., Ordway, G. A., Hauptmann, M., Tejani-Butt, S., Frazer, A. Central administration of 1-isoproterenol *in vivo* induces a

preferential regulation of beta 2-adrenoceptors in the central nervous system of the rat. *Brain Res,* 1991, 555, 141-148.

[88] Reiter, E., Lefkowitz, R. J. GRKs and beta-arrestins: Roles in receptor silencing, trafficking and signaling. *Trends Endocrinol Metab,* 2006, 17, 159-165.

[89] Cervia, D., Martini, D., Ristori, C., Catalani, E., Timperio, A. M., Bagnoli, P., Casini, G. Modulation of the neuronal response to ischaemia by somatostatin analogues in wild-type and knock-out mouse retinas. *J Neurochem,* 2008, 106, 2224-2235.

[90] Hansen, J. L., Theilade, J., Aplin, M., Sheikh, S. P. Role of G-protein-coupled receptor kinase 2 in the heart–do regulatory mechanisms open novel therapeutic perspectives? *Trends Cardiovasc Med,* 2006, 16, 169-177.

[91] Wu, H., Wei, W., Song, L., Zhang, L., Chen, Y., Hu, X. Paeoniflorin induced immune tolerance of mesenteric lymph node lymphocytes via enhancing beta 2-adrenergic receptor desensitization in rats with adjuvant arthritis. *Int Immunopharmacol,* 2007, 7, 662-673.

[92] Krasel, C., Bunemann, M., Lorenz, K., Lohse, M. J. Beta-arrestin binding to the beta2-adrenergic receptor requires both receptor phosphorylation and receptor activation. *J Biol Chem,* 2005, 280, 9528-9535.

[93] Hall, R. A. Beta-adrenergic receptors and their interacting proteins. *Semin Cell Dev Biol,* 2004, 15, 281-288.

[94] Lands, A. M., Arnold, A., McAuliff, J. P., Luduena, F. P., Brown, T. G. Jr. Differentiation of receptor systems activated by sympathomimetic amines. *Nature,* 1967, 214, 597-598.

[95] Emorine, L. J., Marullo, S., Briend-Sutren, M. M., Patey, G., Tate, K., Delavier-Klutchko, C., Strosberg, A. D. Molecular characterization of the human beta3-adrenergic receptor. *Science,* 1989, 245, 1118-1121.

[96] Dessy, C., Balligand, J. L. Beta3-adrenergic receptors in cardiac and vascular tissues emerging concepts and therapeutic perspectives. *Adv Pharmacol* 2010, 59, 1351-1363.

[97] Ursino, M. G., Vasina, V., Raschi, E., Crema, F., de Ponti, F. The beta3-adrenoceptor as a therapeutic target: Current perspectives. *Pharmacological Research,* 2009, 59, 221-234.

[98] Sakane, N., Yoshida, T., Yoshioka, K., Nakamura, Y., Umekawa, T., Kogure, A., Takakura, Y., Kondo, M. Beta 3-adrenoreceptor gene polymorphism: a newly identified risk factor for proliferative retinopathy in NIDDM patients. *Diabetes,* 1997, 46, 1633-1636.

[99] Hoffmann, C., Leitz, M. R., Oberdorf-Maass, S., Lohse, M. J., Klotz, K. N. Comparative pharmacology of human beta-adrenergic receptor subtypes: Characterization of stably transfected receptors in CHO cells. *Naunyn Schmiedebergs Arch Pharmacol,* 2004, 369, 151-159.

[100] Dal Monte, M., Filippi, L., Bagnoli, P. Beta3-adrenergic receptors modulate vascular endothelial growth factor release in response to hypoxia through the nitric oxide pathway in mouse retinal explants. *Naunyn Schmiedebergs Arch Pharmacol,* 2013, 386, 269-278.

[101] Hodis, J., Vaclavikova, R., Farghali, H. Beta-3 agonist-induced lipolysis and nitric oxide production: relationship to PPARgamma agonist/ antagonist and AMP kinase modulation. *Gen Physiol Biophys,* 2011, 30, 90-99.

[102] Massion, P. B., Dessy, C., Desjardins, F., Pelat, M., Havaux, X., Belge, C., Moulin, P., Guiot, Y., Feron, O., Janssens, S., Balligand, J. L. Cardiomyocyte-restricted overexpression of endothelial nitric oxide synthase (NOS3) attenuates beta-adrenergic stimulation and reinforces vagal inhibition of cardiac contraction. *Circulation,* 2004, 110, 2666-2672.

[103] Ignarro, L. J., Sisodia, M., Trinh, K., Bedrood, S., Wu, G., Wei, L. H., Buga, G. M. Nebivolol inhibits vascular smooth muscle cell proliferation by mechanisms involving nitric oxide but not cyclic GMP. *Nitric Oxide,* 2002, 7, 83-90.

[104] Breit, A., Lagacé, M., Bouvier, M. Hetero-oligomerization between beta2- and beta3-adrenergic receptors generates a beta-adrenergic signaling unit with distinct functional properties. *J Biol Chem,* 2004, 279, 28756-28765.

[105] Li, S. Y., Fu, Z. J., Lo, A. C. Y. Hypoxia-induced oxidative stress in ischemic retinopathy. *Oxid Med Cell Longev,* 2012, 2012, 426769.

[106] Van der Wijk, T., Blanchetot, C., den Hertog, J. Regulation of receptor protein-tyrosine phosphatase dimerization. *Methods* 2005, 35, 73-79.

[107] Dal Monte, M., Cammalleri, M., Mattei, E., Filippi, L., Bagnoli, P. Protective effects of β1/2 adrenergic receptor deletion in a model of oxygen-induced retinopathy. *Invest Ophthalmol Vis Sci,* 2015, 56, 59-73.

[108] Witmer, A. N., Vrensen, G. F., Van Noorden, C. J., Schlingemann, R. O. Vascular endothelial growth factors and angiogenesis in eye disease. *Prog Retin Eye Res,* 2003, 22, 1-29.

[109] Olsson, A. K., Dimberg, A., Kreuger, J., Claesson-Welsh, L. VEGF receptor signalling- in control of vascular function. *Nat Rev Mol Cell Biol,* 2006, 7, 359-371.

[110] Filippi, L., Cavallaro, G., Bagnoli, P., Dal Monte, M., Fiorini, P., Donzelli, G., Tinelli, F., Araimo, G., Cristofori, G., la Marca, G., della Bona, M. L., la Torre, A., Fortunato, P., Furlanetto, S., Osnaghi, S., Mosca, F. Oral propranolol for retinopathy of prematurity: risks, safety concerns, and perspectives. *J Pediatr,* 2013, 163, 1570-1577.e6.

[111] Makhoul, I. R., Peleg, O., Miller, B., Bar-Oz, B., Kochavi, O., Mechoulam, H., Mezer, E., Ulanovsky, I., Smolkin, T., Yahalom, C., Khoury, A., Lorber, A., Nir, A., Blazer, S. Oral propranolol versus placebo for retinopathy of prematurity: a pilot, randomised, double-blind prospective study. *Arch Dis Child,* 2013, 98, 565-567.

[112] Filippi, L., Cavallaro, G., Fiorini, P., Daniotti, M., Benedetti, V., Cristofori, G., Araimo, G., Ramenghi, L., la Torre, A., Fortunato, P., Pollazzi, L., la Marca, G., Malvagia, S., Bagnoli, P., Ristori, C., Dal Monte, M., Bilia, A. R., Isacchi, B., Furlanetto, S., Tinelli, F., Cioni, G., Donzelli, G., Osnaghi, S., Mosca, F. Study protocol: safety and efficacy of propranolol in newborns with Retinopathy of Prematurity (PROP-ROP): ISRCTN18523491. *BMC Pediatr,* 2010, 10, 83.

[113] Section on Ophthalmology American Academy of Pediatrics; American Academy of Ophthalmology; American Association for Pediatric Ophthalmology and Strabismus. Screening examination of premature infants for retinopathy of prematurity. *Pediatrics,* 2006, 117, 572-576.

[114] Jalali, S., Balakrishnan, D., Zeynalova, Z., Padhi, T. R., Rani, P. K. Serious adverse events and visual outcomes of rescue therapy using adjunct bevacizumab to laser and surgery for retinopathy of prematurity. The Indian Twin Cities Retinopathy of Prematurity Screening database Report number 5. *Arch Dis Child Fetal Neonatal Ed,* 2013, 98, F327-F333.

[115] Della Bona, M. L., Malvagia, S., Villanelli, F., Giocaliere, E., Ombrone, D., Funghini, S., Filippi, L., Cavallaro G., Bagnoli P., Guerrini R., la Marca, G. A rapid liquid chromatography tandem mass spectrometry-based method for measuring propranolol on dried blood spots. *J Pharm Biomed Anal,* 2013, 78-79, 34-38.

[116] Filippi, L., Cavallaro, G., Fiorini, P., Malvagia, S., della Bona, M. L., Giocaliere, E., Bagnoli, P., Dal Monte, M., Mosca, F., Donzelli, G., la Marca G. Propranolol concentrations after oral administration in term and preterm neonates. *J Matern Fetal Neonatal Med,* 2013, 26, 833-840.

[117] Pieh, C., Krüger, M., Lagrèze, W. A., Gimpel, C., Buschbeck, C., Zirrgiebel, U., Agostini H. T. Plasma sE-selectin in premature infants: a

possible surrogate marker of retinopathy of prematurity. *Invest Ophthalmol Vis Sci,* 2010, 51, 3709-3713.

[118] Raab, S., Beck, H., Gaumann, A., Yüce, A., Gerber, H. P., Plate, K., Hammes, H. P., Ferrara, N., Breier, G. Impaired brain angiogenesis and neuronal apoptosis induced by conditional homozygous inactivation of vascular endothelial growth factor. *Thromb Haemost,* 2004, 91, 595-605.

[119] Haigh, J. J., Morelli, P. I., Gerhardt, H., Haigh, K., Tsien, J., Damert, A., Miquerol, L., Muhlner, U., Klein, R., Ferrara N., Wagner, E. F., Betsholtz, C., Nagy A. Cortical and retinal defects caused by dosage-dependent reductions in VEGF-A paracrine signaling. *Dev Biol,* 2003, 262, 225-241.

[120] Costello, J. M., Franklin, W. H. *Preoperative and postoperative care of the infant with congenital heart disease.* MacDonald, M. G., Seshia, M. M. K., Mullett M. D editors. Avery's neonatology pathophysiology & management of the newborn (6th ed.). Philadelphia: Lippincott Williams & Wilkins; 2005; 738.

[121] University of Wisconsin, Madison. *Propranolol for Diabetic Retinopathy.* 2012. (http://clinicaltrials.gov/show/NCT01535495).

[122] Arevalo, J. F., Arias, J. D., Serrano, M. A. Oral propranolol for exudative retinal detachment in diffuse choroidal hemangioma. *Arch Ophthalmol,* 2011, 129, 1373-1375.

[123] Missoi, T. G., Lueder, G. T., Gilbertson, K., Bayliss, S. J. Oral propranolol for treatment of periocular infantile hemangiomas. *Arch Ophthalmol* 2011, 129, 899-903.

In: Retinopathy of Prematurity (ROP)
Editor: Elmira Aguilar
ISBN: 978-1-63482-644-0

Chapter 2

Retinopathy of Prematurity in the Context with Quality of Life

Kateřina Stejskalová*
Institute of Special Education, Faculty of Education,
Palacky University Olomouc, Czech Republic

Abstract

This text is focused on the area of quality of life for children with retinopathy of prematurity. It deals with retinopathy of prematurity and its influence on the personal experience of the quality of life in the pediatric population. The aim is to illustrate the diverse effects of retinopathy of prematurity on the quality of life of individuals and consequences related to it.

Scientific evaluation of the quality of life is currently phenomenon in the sphere of interest of many disciplines. Efforts to subjective assessment of quality of life is also currently enforced in special education. Quality of life could be characterized by several attributes, which illustrate the current state of scientific knowledge - broad applicability, multidimensional character, vague terminology definition,

* Ph. Dr. Kateřina Stejskalová, Ph. D., Institute of Special Education, Faculty of Education, Palacky University Olomouc, Czech Republic; e-mail: katerina.stejskalova@gmail.com.

distinctive interdisciplinary, diverse interpretability, conceptual fragmentation and multifactorial conditionality. The suggested enumeration eloquently reflects the complexity, variability and lack of clarity of the concept of quality of life. Despite the diversity theoretical points, models, approaches and terminology, common element is conception of human as a bio-psycho-social complex. Emphasis is placed on subjective assessment and its preference before objectively measurable attributes.

Given this fact is emerging a fundamental question - Why should be the quality of life actually explored? Spilker (1990) notes, that at the individual level, answer is obvious - the purpose is to improve individually oriented interventions. Comes to the fore the issue of the quality of life for specific client groups, the aim is an adequate level of support and optimization of complex interventions. In this context arose the concept of quality of life of children with retinopathy of prematurity.

This disease remains the leading cause of childhood blindness in developed and moderately developed countries. Thanks to this is ROP in interest of ophthalmologists worldwide. ROP causes up to 70% of pediatric blindness (Kuchynka et al. 2007). This vazoproliferative retinal disease mainly affects premature infants with low birth weight. Its incidence increases with a percentage of surviving of extremely preterm infants. The spectrum of the resulting anatomical and structural changes and functional consequences is variable, but almost always impaired visual function as a result. New possibilities of therapy with bevacizumab have encouraging results, however ROP and especially its atypical forms remain the focus of experts.

Is clear that the ROP plays an essential role in the development of visual functions - affects early critical period of visual development and is located at key post - on the retina. Even in cases where the ROP regresses spontaneously, there are certain anatomical changes that can secondarily cause visual impairment.

Current scientific and technical progress in medical care, respectively neonatology, perinatology, and especially ophthalmology, significantly improved the prognosis of visual function, even though ROP may have fatal consequences in the form of complete loss of visual perception.

As part of our research, we tried to identify and describe some of the attributes that can specifically determine the quality of life of each individual. Some of the effects of visual impairment can hamper life satisfaction and well-being and may affect the fundamental pillars of quality of life. ROP thus remains the current medical, social, economic and ethical issue.

The aim of qualitatively oriented research was the identification and comprehensive analysis of the specifics of the target group and their depth description. The aim is to optimize intervention process and ideally improve the quality of life of clients. The basic idea is the subjective evaluation of the impact of ROP on the quality of life of the child. One of the objectives of this work is to identify the relevant indicators of quality of life specific to the child population with this type of visual impairment.

In the text is presented theoretical background which make comprehensive theoretical framework for design research. Subsequently are presented outcomes of empirical research, which take the form of primary probe into the selected area.

1. Theoretical Background

Retinopathy of Prematurity, Retinopathia praematurorum ("ROP") is at present on the top of the list of causes of blindness of children in developed countries of the world. This is why it is in the focus of interest of neonatology and ophthalmology experts worldwide. ROP was the cause of eyesight loss for ca 70% of the blind children (Rozsíval, 2005). This vasoproliferative disease of the retina affects especially prematurely born children with low birth weight. Prematurity and the related low birth weight and gestation age present the dominant etiological factors. The ROP incidence grows due to the increasing number of extremely premature children, who manage to survive. In the Czech Republic every year 80% of children with less than 1000 g birth weight survive (Štembera, 2004). Concerning the occurrence of ROP the most risky group are children with birth weight below 1500 g born before the 32nd gestation week (Rozsíval, 2005). Every year in the Czech Republic there are registered ca sixty children with serious damage of vision due to ROP (Kuchynka et al. 2007). The contemporary advances in ophthalmology have significantly improved the prognosis of vision functions of children with ROP, yet its impact can have fatal consequences of total loss of visual perception, which confirms its dominant position among the child blindness causes. The most serious effects of ROP affect 10-30% children with this disease (Kuchynka et al. 2007).

The presented data clearly show, that ROP remains, in spite of the significant scientific and technical advances in neonatology and ophthalmology care, a very pressing medical, social, economic, social-pedagogic and ethical problem. Depending from the level of retained eyesight functions, which range from weak eyesight up to total blindness and in connection with other accompanying complications arising from the degree of immaturity, there was prepared a concept focusing on the quality of life of children, who suffer from retinopathy of prematurity.

The most frequent effect of ROP is serious eyesight impairment, or even blindness. ROP is at the top of the list of the most frequent causes of child blindness in medium developed and advanced countries. Due to the technical advances in the neonatology and perinatology fields we can expect rising incidence in the category of extremely immature newborns at the very limit of viability, which will mean a rising incidence of retinopathy of prematurity, especially its atypical forms. It is these atypical forms, which are the most typical of significant anatomical changes with a fatal impact on the eyesight functions.

The loss of vision affects the whole personality of an individual and his/her quality of life. According to the degree of eyesight loss the individual suffers from various degrees of information deficit and the information perception becomes distorted. Most of information people get is of visual nature, so the lowered visual perception creates an information barrier, which needs to be compensated with alternative mechanisms. In this context there is highlighted the need to use compensation and rehabilitation aids in order to maximally use the existing vision potential. The limitation is reflected also in limited ability to use the ordinary black print, usually significant enlargement of font is needed and in the ultimate cases the text must be transcribed into Braill. Damage of eyesight functions affects the quality of perception of depth and space, ability to localise, analyse, synthesise or the ability of visual-motoric coordination, the level of which is significantly limited. If a person is born with damaged eyesight, or if eyesight is lost at an early age, the development of cognitive and learning processes is also affected and disturbed, such as formation of imagination, memory, thinking and speech. Due to insufficient quantity or total loss of visual stimuli for a person born with damaged eyesight, sensory deprivation may be manifested. This can be positively affected by timely re-education of the remaining eyesight, if any, and especially by the development of compensating senses, especially touch and hearing in interaction with other, higher compensation mechanisms (Růžičková, 2006).

The decisive factor for a successful development of the remaining eyesight functions and the compensating elements is timely diagnostics and appropriate expert intervention, which can partially alleviate the sensual deprivation.

The QOL (Quality of Life) phenomenon is an issue, which is currently highly discussed and widely understood and many fields of science study it (philosophy, sociology, psychology, medicine, economy, ecology, pedagogy, special pedagogy etc.). Of course, each of these fields adopts a specific viewing angle, which brings out different theoretical starting points. The wide options of application are reflected in the multi dimensional nature of this problematic. The wide applicability can be seen in the multidimensional nature of this issue. The interest in quality of life is not a modern trend – its roots trace back to Greek and Roman mythology and the recent interest can be dated back to the 30's of the 20th century if the concept of quality of life can be said to have been introduced in the sphere of psychology (Mühlpacher, Vaďurová, 2006). The World Health Organization defines the quality of life as the individual's perception of his role in life in the context of his culture and value system, in relation to his goals, expectations, standards and concerns. It is a wide concept multifactorially conditioned by physical health, mental state, personal confession, social relations and relation to the key areas of his environment (Vaďurová, 2006).

The assessment of QOL of children has become the focus of interest of experts only during the last ten years. A wide range of research is dedicated to the quality of life of the adult population, however the category of children and adolescents is slowly gaining in importance and it becomes an "emerging field of study." In the past there were developed various theories describing the quality of life of children. Mostly the theories focused on only one dominant aspect of a child's world. According to the present view of many authors, the development theories focusing on the psychological aspect (e.g. Limber, Hashima, 1999), or physical aspect (such as Ruštin, Greenberg, 1999), social (e.g. Flakkoy, Hevener, 1997), moral or spiritual growth (such as Thompson, Randal, 1999) do not provide sufficiently complex basis for creation of tools to monitor QOL of children (Dostálek, Troneček, Hejcmanová, Petriščáková in Mareš et al. 2006). Currently even in this area of interest there dominate the quantitative methods of QOL assessment in the form of questionnaires, which may not be sufficiently sensitive to the specifics of certain groups of children, especially ill children. The questionnaires are also designed for an "average" child, which does not exist. This is why there is a worldwide increase of interest in a qualitative approach and specific instruments of qualitative nature (Mareš, Marešová in Koukola, Mareš, 2007).

From another perspective, the aforesaid authors speak about other problematic aspects of measuring the quality of life of children – we, the adults, ask children from our point of view, using our methods and our words. Vaďurová (2006) notes the attention span and points out, that in reasonable cases there is no other alternative than "proxy rating," when the quality of life is assessed by a parent, doctor or other relative.

This brings us to the question of the evaluator of the quality of life. Vaďurová (2006) considers the assessment of the source of information as a very important aspect of the QOL assessment. The source of information may be the patients (clients), nurses, medical staff. Each of the groups clearly provides a different point of view about the quality of life of a child and interprets the situation from its own perspective. One of the variants is the "proxy rating" - assessment done by the parent or nurse. The parent's opinion about the quality of life of a child may not be quite relevant, it may be distorted for instance due to different perception of the present situation of the child and anticipation of its future and it can be significantly determined by emotional influences. In this context Salajka (2006) notes, that the tools assessing the HRQOL of children have until recently almost always been based on data from the relatives, usually the mother.

Measurement of the quality of life of disabled children may be even more complicated. QOL of specific client groups must be assessed so we could improve the quality and optimise the complex individualised intervention in order to achieve the maximum possible social integration of a handicapped person into the intact society. Even in this context the total QOL cannot be described only by health indicators. An illustration of this is the definition of health created by the National Institute on Disability and Rehabilitation Research - "Being handicapped does not equal being ill." The medicine model defines handicap as a problem primarily caused by an illness or other situation, which requires medical intervention, which is a solution to the problem. The international classification of functioning, handicap and health according to WHO on the other hand emphasises the social dimension of a handicap and the limitations arising from that (Vaďurová, Mühlpachr, 2005). In the recent decades there has been spreading an attitude, that the handicapped people themselves identify the elements of the "disabling environment" instead of the axiom, that the organic damage is the primary source of their problems. This has led to a significant change of paradigm, when the functional limitation was replaced with a model of a minority group, which faces basically the same problems as other disadvantaged groups (Hahn in Vaďurová, 2006).

1.1. Excursus into the Issue of Prematurity

It is significant that this chapter "born" together with the theme of preterm, premature newborns. Due to increasing quality of care and scientific progress in the field of neonatology and perinatology, the issue is becoming increasingly important. It is characterized by fundamental economic and ethical dimension. Recent developments in neonatology significantly improved the prognosis of prematurity, or extremely preterm infants. Despite this fact arise from such life circumstances often very significant long-term complications, often lifelong.

In response to the increasing incidence of extremely preterm infants can be expected also a rising incidence of people with visual impairment due to retinopathy of prematurity, despite the current possibilities of the ophthalmologic care. Currently Czech neonatal mortality is one of the lowest in the world. Every year survived around 80% of infants weighing less than 1000 grams. The incidence of this category of newborns increased from 0.15% in 1989 to 0.35% today, which is comparable to the incidence of developed countries (Štembera, 2004).

In this context, it is still intensively discussed issue of determining the boundaries of viability. At our country and abroad is recognized boundary finished 24th week of pregnancy. Retinopathy of prematurity is one of the complications of extreme immaturity and has major economic, medical and ethical dimensions and becomes an interdisciplinary subject of concern in several of disciplines focusing to human.

Prematurity is associated with a relatively broad spectrum of health complications, the incidence and severity is directly commensurate with the degree of immaturity of the newborn. One major problem is respiratory distress, the cause of which is immature lung tissue and the absence of surfactant. Immature structure of lung tissue reduced alveolar surface and a lack of lung surfactant leads to an RDS (respiratory distress syndrome), which threaten the child with respiratory failure (Roztočil et al. 2008). RDS arises from the immaturity of the lung, due to which there is insufficient exchange of respiratory gases. Neonatal RDS is then cause of situation in which each breath is as demanding as the first, requiring high pressure to reopen collapsed alveoli (Dickason, Silverman, Schult, 1994).

In the context of breathing problems are frequent apnea and bradycardia accompanied by cyanosis (Leifer, 2004). Difficulties can arise in thermogenesis and thermoregulation - due to absence of protective insulating layer of subcutaneous fat and poor thermoregulation may cause hypothermia. Also hypoglycemia and hypocalcemia can complicate the health status of newborn leading to brain damage. Another problematic aspect is nutrition and hydration in terms of poor sucking, swallowing, bowel motility and low production of digestive enzymes.

After the big loss of blood during childbirth, due to infection and most often as a result of immaturity adrenal hormonal responses to stress with hypotension may occur. Due to accelerated decay of erythrocytes in combination with reduced haemopoiesis is often manifested anemia. As a consequence of immature hepatic functions might occur to hyperbilirubinemia (Fendrychová, Borek et al. 2007). Threatens an increased risk of skin damage that is immature and fragile (Fendrychová, Borek et al. 2007).

Also kidneys are affected by functional immaturity. There are problems with the maintenance of homeostatic mechanisms, tendency to edema, hyponatremia, hypokalemia and acidosis. Complications may even result in kidney failure. Significantly is affected the immune system. Morphological and functional immaturity is the basis of physiological immunodeficiency premature newborn, which is manifested by frequent infections and severe sepsis with high mortality (Roztočil et al. 2008).

Other complications include acute necrotizing enterocolitis or enteritis leading to necrosis (Leifer, 2004). The digestive system also related to complicated nutrition - the capacity of the stomach is very small, at both ends of the sphincter of the stomach are immature and it leads to vomiting during feeding. Immature sucking and swallowing reflexes limited the ability to absorb fats and fat-soluble vitamins. Due to above characteristics is a clear need for a feeding gavage or parenterally. Parenteral nutrition is one of the cornerstones of comprehensive care for critically ill or premature newborn.

A one of the most common of difficulties is postnatal adaptation. Is constitute from a series adaptive changes - physiological, biochemical, immunological and hormonal aiming to adapting the newborn extrauterine environment. Zoban (in Fuchs, Zoban et al. 2001) emphasizes that these newborns require a specialized and often intensive care because they are not prepared to adaptation seamlessly to the conditions of an ectopic environment.

At the conclusion of this section, it is necessary to mention the effects of prematurity on visual functions. In addition to the most serious complications of prematurity, which is ROP, there may be other serious limits of visual perception. A study of Larsson et al. (2005) demonstrated that in premature infants is high prevalence of visual and neurological disorders. Also have been revealed significant differences in visual function in preterm infants (ten years old) compared with a control group of children born in normal time. The results show a higher incidence of reduced visual acuity in preterm.

In the group of infants born before 28 weeks of gestation was Spencer (2006) reported 4,1 times higher risk of abnormal visual acuity compared with infants born after the 28th week of pregnancy. In children with generally poorer health related to prematurity we can record 5,3 times higher risk of abnormal visual acuity. Long-term development of visual functions in extremely premature infants with very low birth weight is proven to be associated with a high risk of deterioration of visual acuity - the highest risk group includes children born before 28 weeks of gestation.

1.2. Eye Findings Associated with ROP

The population of children with spontaneous regression of ROP is characterized by increased incidence of specific visual defects. In this category we find a significantly increased proportion of strabism (14-40%), nystagmus (16-50%) and amblyopia (6-33%) compared with the category of infants born in term (Rozsíval et al. 2005). Also other authors confirm this risk category for the occurrence of subsequent ophthalmological complications, to which also includes the late retinal detachment, glaucoma and myopia (in the incidence of around 10%) (Bashour, 2008).

Odehnal, Filouš (1998) further specify that a higher percentage of refractive errors, particularly myopia, strabism and pseudostrabism is characteristic concomitant of mild forms of ROP. During course of severe ROP occurs secondary glaucoma, complicated cataract, corneal dystrophic changes and late traction retinal detachment. Zobanová (2005) to the other long term complications associated with ROP assigns ptosis, anterior segment changes, fluctuations in intraocular pressure, macular degeneration, the formation of vitreoretinal proliferation or atrophy of the eyeball. In pubescence also increases the risk of late retinal detachment.

The most severe anatomical and structural consequences of ROP affect approximately 10-30% of children with this disease. Currently also increases incidence of atypical forms of ROP with an unfavorable prognosis.

2. Underlying Ideas of the Research

The quality of life issues can be defined by several attributes, which illustrate the contemporary state of scientific research in this area - wide applicability, multi-dimensional nature, vague terminology, strong interdisciplinary overlaps, differing interpretations, fragmented concepts and multifactor conditionality. In spite of a great diversity in the theoretical background, models, approaches and terminology, the unifying element is the attempt to present a complex view of a person on various levels, which reflect the overall quality of life with an accent on the subjective feelings and the person's preferences instead of objectively measurable attributes.

Apart from the anatomical-functional changes connected with ROP, the key actor is the psycho-social dimension of the eyesight impairment caused by it. We consider this dimension of the eyesight impairment as an axis for the assessment of the quality of life. In this sense we attempted to identify and describe some of the attributes, which participate in the formation of the subjectively perceived quality of life significantly and determine it, specifically in integration with other factors.

The theoretical background of special education of children with visual impairment still suffers from the absence of relevant research studies. The objective of our research was to enrich and widen the theoretical foundations of special education of children with visual impairment, which should reflect the latest scientific findings about this issue. On the practical level it should lead to the maximum possible individualisation and optimisation of special pedagogy intervention for this category of individuals. The main goal of the research was subjective evaluation of the ROP impact on the quality of life of individuals, with the focus on child population. One of the partial objectives was to identify relevant QOL indicators specific for children with this type of visual impairment. Due to the present state of knowledge about ROP we still do not have sufficient knowledge about its impact on the quality of life. It can be expected that due to the rising incidence of newborns in the category of extremely immature and the related occurrence of ROP, the need for a deeper description of the specifics of this category will be emphasised more and more. The key objective of our work was to open door for the related applied research.

A similar issue - the evaluation of the quality of life related to health in the category of 10 year-old children with a very low birth weight with the threshold phase of the ROP and without it - was dealt with, but from a different perspective, by the American authors Quinn, Dobson, Saigal and others. For the evaluation of the quality of life they used the Health Utilities Index System reflecting 8 areas: vision, hearing, talking, walking, dexterity, emotions, cognitive functions, and pain. (Available at http://archopht.ama-assn.org/cgi/content/abstract/122/11/1659). This study was focused in particular on the aspects of health condition and physical health. To compare, the research we anticipate to make will be conceived as wide-spectrum -

including, in particular, the subjectively problematic areas of the quality of life related to the given category of individuals with ROP.

3. Survey Design

Though the present dominant trend is to use quantitative methods to measure QOL, such as generic and specific questionnaires, the presented research is conceived as qualitative. So far the experts have not clearly solved the question, how can quality of life be assessed quantitatively and to what extent the used questionnaires are suitable for this purpose. In the context of the target group of our survey there is also the specific and so far not scientifically preferred field of QOL measurement of children, modified for children with health disability, often combined with other disabilities.

Not only due to the aforesaid factors the worldwide interest in the qualitative methods and qualitative approach as such is rising. We decided to reflect this trend and conceive a qualitative design for our survey. Due to the character of the researched subset we consider qualitative methods as the most relevant.

Mareš (in Mareš et al. 2006) characterises qualitative approach to QOL assessment as an approach, which does not attempt precision and generalisation. The author (2006) also notes, that these methods rely on semi-standardised interview with an individual and try to understand his or her personal (often unique) life experience. Qualitative methods in general enrich our view of the examined problem and allow us to generate new hypotheses.

Svatoš, Švarcová (in Mareš et al. 2006) point out to methodological difficulty, when a child subjectively assesses the quality of its own life – unlike adults here it is methodologically more difficult to get reliable data about quality of life from a self assessment - especially in case of little children, in general it can be said, that with falling age our diagnostic options decrease. This is one of the reasons for combining a subjective self-assessment performed by children with ROP and proxy rating provided by parents or nurses.

Due to the problematic aspects connected with the assessment of QOL of children with vision impairment, the chosen data acquisition method is semi-structured interview, which should reflect the aforesaid problematic nuances so the interpretation imprecision is as reduced as possible. At the same time this method should contribute to a truly subjective assessment of the child's life quality and it should allow for identification of the subjectively important elements of the child's everyday life.

4. Interpretation of the Research Outcomes

Our survey should help as a primary research about the development of children with ROP. At the same time we would like to point out that the given results and their interpretation must always be interpreted locally in the given context – we did not attempt generalisation for wider population, since generalisation can be made only upon a theory. The result is an integrative description based on authentic opinions and statements of the respondents, so we could paint a maximally complex picture about the life experiences of children with ROP in the context of their quality of life. The purpose was to illustrate the sensitive indicators important for the individual perspective and the overall quality of life. During the realisation of the survey, among others based on the study of domestic and foreign peer review literature, we chose the following research questions, whereas some of them emerged spontaneously from the data only during the very research:

- What are the characteristics of the quality of life with retinopathy of prematurity?
- In what way does retinopathy of prematurity affect the quality of life of children?
- What is the subjective perception of the quality of life of children with retinopathy of prematurity?
- Is retinopathy of prematurity subjectively viewed as something connected with worse quality of life?
- What areas of quality of life are considered by children with retinopathy of prematurity as subjectively problematic, or which are the most determined by eyesight impairment?
- How do children with retinopathy of prematurity view their quality of life and how does their view differ from the one of their parents?
- What is the role of the overall health condition in the assessment of the quality of life of children with retinopathy of prematurity?

Concerning the first of the research questions (*What are the characteristics of the quality of life with retinopathy of prematurity?*) our objective was to define the individually specific and subjectively assessed level of the quality of life. At the same time we wanted to define the specific predictors of QOL improvement based on identification of any specific indicators.

We proposed such indicators we consider relevant - they reflect all the three aforesaid dimensions and thus they allow to fully capture the characteristics of the quality of life of each individual. The preparation of the tools to measure the QOL of children with ROP was based especially on the comparison of standardised generic QOL questionnaires from WHO and other specific questionnaires for child clients and for the population with eyesight impairment.

Though we used general measurement instruments to create the concept of the assessed QOL areas, the tool we designed can be considered as adequately sensitive. The spectrum of indicators corresponds to the empirically verified areas of QOL of the intact population, so we can expect that it captures all the relevant attributes. Schalock (2009, p. 5) confirms our approach on a more general level: "Individual quality of life is a multidimensional phenomenon consisting of key areas affected by both personality and environment. These key areas are the same for all humans, though they may differ individually according to the relative value and importance." The general measurement instruments thus reflect even specific indicators for the category of people with visual impairment, who however have different individually specific characteristics. Due to a relatively wide range of the used indicators, they can be expected to cover all the subjectively important aspects of the quality of life. At the same time the assessed indicators are identical with the determining factors of the quality of life of each individual, regardless the existence of any health problems. However the resulting profile of the quality of life bears the specific characteristics of a disability, in this case a visual disability.

The second of the presented research questions (*In what way does retinopathy of prematurity affect the quality of life of children?*) has a very wide scope - from individually specific characteristics of health condition - concerning the retained vision functions there are two extreme positions, when comparing the case studies and authentic interviews - through other anamnesis data confirming the aforesaid variability of the overall health condition; up to the characteristics of mental and social dimension related to the visual or even combined disability. Authentic statements, or individual QOL profiles allowed us to capture and describe all the differences in the individually specific quality of life indicators.

These aspects can be further connected with the interpretation of results related to the third and fourth question (*What is the subjective perception of the quality of life of children with retinopathy of prematurity? Is retinopathy of prematurity subjectively assessed as something connected with worse quality of life?*). It is clear, that ROP and complications connected with prematurity affect the quality of life. On the individual level, the question is how to determine the subjectively perceived well-being. International research concerning the quality of life of people with disabilities examined a representative sample and proved specific features identified by a wide range of disabled people - a communication and information barrier between the intact population and the community of the disabled, which has implications for social integration, acceptance and non-acceptance by the intact society and also identification with the community of the disabled. These characteristics are, due to the age range of the respondents, especially in the casuistic studies made by us.

Though it is not possible to reach a truly relevant generalisation, there is no denying, that ROP significantly determines the quality of visual perception and secondarily even the whole development of an individual concerning the possible strong vision impairment with all the described negative impacts and limitations. Another complication is the etiology factor of the ROP formation - prematurity implying a number of health complications, often life endangering, and late polymorbidity. The above mentioned attributes certainly contribute to the personal well-being and in the general sense they affect the quality of life of each individual.

The generally accepted view is that health disability implies a lower quality of life, however regardless the resulting health condition, which may or may not be affected by these factors, we would like to highlight an empirical confirmation of the "disability paradox" which brings also one of answers to the fourth research question (*Is retinopathy of prematurity subjectively viewed as something connected with worse quality of life?*) - it is a disparity between the objectively documented serious diagnosis and its expected serious impact as viewed by the exterior evaluators on one side and the subjectively positive evaluation of quality of life by the persons, who lives with health problems (Mareš, Marešová in Řehulka, Řehulková, Blatný, Mareš et al. 2008). Mareš, Marešová (in Řehulka, Řehulková, Blatný, Mareš et al. 2008) call it a paradox of the beneficial influence of health problems.

The research of this phenomenon has shown, that people with various types of health problems claim to have the same or even higher quality of life than people, who are healthy or "intact." So we cannot a priori anticipate a lowered quality of life, even though serious scientific studies (Silva, Oliveira, Ferreira, Pereira, 2005) proved a significant impact of health impairment on the quality of life of an individual - as we have emphasised several times, in case of QOL it is a multifactor conditioned concept, which needs not necessarily be affected by health condition, or the limits arising from it. The authors also present an explanation for this divergence, as shown by Albrecht and Devlieger (in Řehulková, Řehulka, Blatný, Mareš et al. 2008, p. 11) using the theory of balance: "Many people with a serious disease can find a balance among the physical, mental and spiritual segment of their lives. They are helped also by the positive influence of their environment, whether it is social or nature environment." This explanation can be applied also to the problem of health or visual disability. An illustration can be found in the casuistic study of Lukáš, based on which we can predict good quality of life and especially positive development towards a self-supporting, independent and satisfied life. Our findings are more optimistic, than we had anticipated originally, not only concerning the retained visual functions, but also concerning the assessment of the overall development and the related social factors. In this context Salajka (2006) points to a very careful and reasonable interpretation of the data acquired from the QOL assessment. Also, considering the disability paradox, he warns about the possibility of data distortion due to the prejudice, which automatically expects the health problems to have a negative impact on the quality of life. In this sense he highlights the individual hierarchy of life values, the level of adaptability to changed conditions and the ability to "perceive various aspects, which form the rich tapestry of everyday life, to what extent this influence will manifest, how much it is perceived by the ill person" (Salajka, 2006, p. 105). On the level of the third research question (*What is the subjective perception of the quality of life of children with retinopathy of prematurity?*), apart from the aforesaid disability paradox we can only highlight the individually specific profiles of the quality of life of each respondent, including the case studies, their multifactor conditionality in a specific authentic context.

Of all the proposed indicators of the quality of life, the most highlighted one - not only by our respondents - is the psycho-social dimension, which is - in compliance with the outcomes of the international handicapped person QOL assessment projects - the main troublesome dimension of a disability - which opens the question of the attitude of the intact population to disabled persons, the question of social integration, influence of the disability on the process of socialisation of an individual, the level of acceptance and non-acceptance of the handicap and identification with the community of the handicapped people and a number of other long term topical all-society issues - the influence of family and the upbringing attitudes of parents, social determinants (wider environment, other members of the same age group, contact with the community of the disabled) and other nuances. On this level we have actually answered the fifth question (*What areas of quality of life are considered by children with retinopathy of prematurity as subjectively problematic, or which are the most determined by eyesight impairment?*). Except the clear value of the authentic reactions, the other aspects of this area are in detail characterised in the respective chapter of the theoretical section of this work dedicated to the impacts of visual impairment.

Concerning the sixth research question (*How do children with retinopathy of prematurity view their quality of life and how does their view differ from the one of their parents?*), there was assessed the hypothetically different viewing angle of the parent and the child about the ROP impact and the related QOL aspects. From the view of the researcher the parents were able to adequately and relative rationally assess the impact of the health problems and the disability on the life of the child. The realised interview also allowed them to reflect on the development of the child and to get a feedback. Schalock (2009) points out, that except providing the feedback there are also other ways, how the data can be useful for the parents - it can create their expectation that change is possible and it can occur on several levels. At the same time it confirms functionality of organisations in the sense of a holistic attitude to the client and comparison of the subjective and objective dimension. In this context it also clarifies the importance of the use of personal data, either in the form of individual or summary information on the organisational level - it highlights the need to allow sharing of information about the client's outcomes and changes on various levels of support, to incorporate the information about the outcomes and the findings arising from that to the theory of scientific disciplines, and last but not least, to define the individual, organisational and community factors, which may indicate the prospective development.

The specific features of the health care of the surveyed group usually have the attributes of a combined disability in the ROP context and also complications connected with prematurity, however some of the contacted respondents feel only minimum negative impact of the aforesaid factors. The level of retained visual functions seems relatively positive in this respondent group, compared with the anamnesis data from the case studies. In the sense of the last research question (*What is the role of the overall health condition in the assessment of the quality of life of children with retinopathy of prematurity?*) we can, again, only point to the individually variable influence on the quality of life.

Concerning the visual impairment and its negative impacts on the independent and his/her well-being, the answer to the last question is clear - if the outcomes of ROP reach the dimension of visual impairment, the psycho-social indicators of QOL are modified in the above presented way.

As part of a specific module intended only for the parents, there was assessed not only QOL of their children in the sense of proxy rating, but we were also interested in the attitudes, feelings and knowledge of the parents concerning the options for the optimal development of the child. Again, we cannot reach a relevant conclusion with an adequate value, but in a number of specific examples we noted very rational democratic approach of the upbringing. However talking about the acceptance of the disability by the parents or by their children, proved to be embarrassing for the parents, as well as the topic of the options to identify with a group of disabled people in order to form an adequate identity of a disabled person this issue of course has implication for the area of personal self-perception, but in a wider dimension also to the social integration area. From the interviews and the casuistic studies we can see an emphasised role of the family and family influence towards adequate socialisation, or social integration and the overall psycho-social dimension of the disability.

In general, our research aimed to become the first survey of a "new or complex area" and initiated a quantitative research while proposing measurement procedures or acquiring a deeper insight into the specifics (Hendl, www.kpg.zcu.cz/capv/HTML/5/5.pdf, p. 5). Our objective was not to create a generalising theory, but to provide a relatively complex picture of the quality of life of children with ROP so as to allow subsequent deep analysis of a quantitative nature.

We based our survey on the concept of capturing the individual life experiences of children with ROP, whereas we did not strive a priori to create any specific generalising theory. Instead we intended to provide a primary insight into the life of children with this diagnosis and to capture the specifics on everyday life level. The individual presented profiles of QOL and casuistic studies of children with ROP should illustrate the nature of limitations concerning the individual QOL indicators, whereas the subjective view was preferred over objectively measurable attributes.

5. Conclusion

What was the premise of our work, from what idea did the research design originated? These questions have been answered in the previous text, however, several characteristics will serve here for final balancing:

- Quality of life - multidimensional, broadly interpreted, multifactiorially conditioned scientific concept attracting in the last three decades attention of expert public within the intentions of social disciplines.
- Retinopathy of the premature babies (ROP) - one of the main causes of sightlessness of children in the economically developed world, a specific disease characteristic for premature babies with low birth weight, which may and, at the same time, due to technological advance in the field of interventional procedures, does not have to lead to fatal consequences in the form of meaning loss of sight perception, respectively to sight disability.
- Extreme immaturity of a new born baby - factor carrying along a very wide spectrum of life threatening complications and late consequences, situations evoking a number of ethical dilemmas, key etiological factor of origin of ROP.
- Sight disability - attribute determining overall development of an individual, factor conditioning the socialization process and social integration process, one of key determinants of quality of life and the life satisfaction.

We decided to reflect these phenomena of contemporary scientific research on various levels of knowledge - the result is a concept of evaluation of quality of life of infant population with ROP with accent on subjective evaluation of impact of above presented factors, mutual interaction of which and determination of complexly understood quality of life in the sense of well-being - personal well being integrating in itself indicators of psychical and social health.

The objective of the research has been to formulate subjective influence and impacts of ROP onto the sphere of regular everyday life and the rate which determines its quality. We tried to evaluate to which extent ROP, and its consequences and other related aspects, influence the quality of life - physical and psychical state, way of life and the feeling of life satisfaction.

Respectively we wanted to confirm empirically correlations between its consequences and altered quality of life. A partial objection was in this matter to find subjective importance and meaning of proposed indicators of quality of life for target group, while, at the same time, identifying other subjectively important factors. In this sense an analysis of the statements of children was a premise. The subject to measurement of quantitative nature was a category of children with ROP, whose current quality of life was evaluated.

The proposed indicators are, according to our opinion, relevant in relation to studied issues and, at the same time, these are identical with the determinants of quality of life of each individual despite the presence of the health disability. However, the resulting profile of quality of life carries just the specific features of health disability, in our case sight disability in particular. Despite it is not possible to reach really relevant evaluation, it is evident that ROP significantly determines quality of sight perception and secondary the entire development of an individual in the sense of potential severe sight disability with all described negative consequences and limitations. As another complication factor comes to the front line the etiological factor of occurrence of ROP - prematurity implicating a number of health, often life threatening, complications and late polymorbidity. The outlined features are undoubtedly taking part in the feeling of personal well-being in the most general sense of the word these influence quality of life of every individual. However, without taking into account the health state, which may or may not be influenced by these described factors, we would like to stress the empiric proof of, so called, disability paradox - illustrating case may be case study of Lukas, on the basis of which we may predict his positive future development towards self-reliant, independent and satisfactory life. Of all the proposed indicators of quality of life psychosocial dimension is accented, not only by our respondents. It is in line with the conclusions of international projects evaluating quality of life of persons with disability, the main acrid dimension of disability - here comes a question of the approach of intact population towards the persons with disabilities, The area of social integration, influence of disability on the socializing process of socialization of an individual, level of acceptation and not acceptation of disability and identifying with a community of persons with disability and a number of others long term topical society-wide topics.

The results of empiric research would, in ideal case, be reflected in optimizing of special pedagogy intervention process with the observed category of individuals with sight disability - both on individual levels, towards improved quality of the approach of professionals, and on the level of organizations in the sense of interdisciplinary cooperation. An integral part of this requisite represents enrichment of theoretical base of special pedagogy of person with sight disability by the phenomenon of the quality of life and especially by the problems of ROP, to which adequate, and from the point of view increasing incidence ever more accenting, attention has not been paid so far. We expect that applicable potential of the research output may be found not only in the field of social pedagogy, but also in medicine, respectively in neonatology and ophthalmology practice. The presented proposals for practice aim also to this conclusion. At the same time the resulting findings may project into the process of creating of a standardized specific tool for measuring the quality of life for the category of persons with ROP. In association to this was one of partial objections checking the extent of proposed concept of evaluating of quality of life of children with this specific disease on a relatively small group and its viability and its use for further applied research.

In general approach our research sought primary acknowledgement "with a new and complicated field of science" and initiation of quantitative research "with proposal of measuring procedures or reaching of deeper insight into peculiarities" (Hendl, www.kpg.zcu.cz/capv/HTML/5/5.pdf, p. 5).

Our objection was not to establish a generalizing theory, but rather to present a relatively complex picture of life of children with ROP.

The key objection of this work was to broaden theoretical base of special pedagogy for persons with sight disability on the basis of longitudinal quality oriented research by, so far never reflected, issues of quality of life of persons with ROP and to open space for related applied research. Secondarily, these efforts should lead to optimizing of complexly understood intervention towards the given target group.

On individual level our objection was not only to present particular life histories, but, at the same time, using this self-evaluation secondarily provide to respondents, respectively to their parents, a feedback, opportunity for self-reflection. On the level of cooperation with professionals should these features, related from distribution of information, to adequacy of approach of experts, and the level of empathy, via interdisciplinary cooperation as far as optimized accessibility of services on various levels, illustrate a very real picture of used services, which should be a premise for further applied research aiming towards saturation of specific needs of individuals with sight disability resulting from ROP and towards increased quality of their everyday life. The pivot point of this idea is achievement of independent, self-reliant and satisfied life on various levels in the sense of well-being.

Conclusion of this work is not based on rough scores or statistical data, not even on generalized theory - it is based on description of images of particular authentic life histories of children with ROP.

6. Illustrative Outputs of the Study

In the following section of text partial outputs of qualitative oriented research will be presented, with respect to extensiveness not only of data management, but of the complex analysis and interpretation of data, we list only illustrative fragments of qualitative data analysis

Table 1. Found features of health diagnosis of respondents in original research file

Health complication	Occurrence	Occurrence in %
ADHD	2	10
Amaurosa	9	45
Amblyopia	2	10
Astigmatism	8	40
Atrophy of papillae n. o.	1	5
Autism	2	10
DMO	7	35
Ectopic macula	1	5
Epilepsy	1	5
Hypermetropia	4	20
Mental retardation	1	5
Myopia	4	20
Nystagmus	3	15
Strabism	4	20

Table 2. Resulting state of sight functions in the original research life

Level of sight disability	Occurrence	Occurrence in %
Blindness	11	55
Purblindness	4	20
Binocular sight disorder	4	20
Sight perception within standard	2	10

6.1. Case Study

Eliška

Date of birth: 11/1/2001
Current age: 9.3 years

Family Anamnesis

Nuclear family consists of four members: mother Kateřina (1976), by occupation optician; father Petr (1966), by occupation car mechanic; both parents have basic education. Sister (twin) Tereza - without sight disability, only light astigmatism diagnosed. In the beginning the parents did not show much interest in services of SPC, the cooperation was rather reserved, employees of the consulting center interpreted it in the beginning as "careful." Currently the cooperation and communication are on a very good level, however the interest of parents in common activities with sight disabled remains low, and it could, to a certain extent, represent an obstacle in acceptance of disability and acceptance of adequate identity - in this respect it is necessary to develop contact with the community of coevals with sight disability towards identification with this category of people. The family lives in a family house near a district town. The parents strive for best possible development of all Eliška´s potential so as for her to be able to succeed in competitive environment of intact society. Their educative approach has perfectionist characteristics, nevertheless, democratic tuning prevails. Parents are heavily concentrated on school performance; Eliška is strongly motivated by their attitude. Family governing has a very positive impact on Eliška´s overall development. In the beginning the family did not see specifics and consequences of sight disability - still the parents gradually adapted a more realistic approach, they also start to support mutual contact - with intact group of coevals and with coevals with sight disability. Nevertheless, the attitudes of parents still imply not acceptance of sight disability. Cooperation with school consultancy office is very good, helpful and the parents are very responsive.

Personal Anamnesis

The mother was due to risk of premature delivery kept in hospital for three months prior to delivery. Eliška was born in week 27 of gestation; the birth was performed by cesarean. With respect to extreme prematurity (birth weight 900 grams) she was kept in an incubator. In the beginning the nutrition was delivered parenterally, eventually by a probe, she was fed by accumulated mother's milk, she was breast fed from 3rd month up to 3 years of age. Due to occurrence of potential complications related to extreme prematurity a series of ophthalmologic and neurological examinations followed. Probably in 6th postnatal week cryocoagulation of retina on both eyes for threshold stadium of ROP was performed – the effect of the surgery was negative, sight functions are within the zone of practical blindness, sense of light remains. The resulting diagnosis ROP IV b - V, partial amotio retinae.

After enrolling to a preschool institution increased sickness rate was observed, other than that Eliška suffered no injuries.

Not strong laterality was diagnosed with Eliška. Mental requisites are in the above average zone - output is stabile across subtests.

Psychomotor Development

From the point of view of psychomotor development retardation was found with Eliška (due to prematurity and sight disability it is standard). Specific was the absence of crawling. Walking occurred in the age of three. In ontogenesis of speech the retardation was not measurable - first words came before she concluded her first year.

Characteristics of Further Development (Educational Process, Cooperation with Specialists, Family Context, Socializing Process, Features of Personality)

Eliška is very sociable, active, curious, approachable and patient, she can be independent. Since 2005 Eliška has been a client of SPC for sight disabled persons. That year she started to attend kindergarten in her place of residence for 4 hours a day. Eliška enrolled into preschool institution for her integration – it was a small village kindergarten. Eliška was educated on the basis of IVP, which was continuously upgraded (in monthly intervals) by a teacher in the kindergarten and it was supervised by employees of SPC. Eliška got adapted to the environment in the kindergarten very quickly. It was rather easy for her to incorporate herself into a group of 17 children, which fact may have been influenced by presence of her twin sister. Eliška established contact with her mates very quickly, she became emancipated and symbolic bond to mother was overcome; tie to the sister was overcome too. She was taking part in all activities of the class. The group and the pedagogues accepted Eliška very well.

The teacher in the preschool institution was trained in issues of education of individuals with sight disability in the form of a seminar organized by SPC.

SPC also provided necessary methodological support and aid and other services in the sense of lending of specialized literature and aids. From the point of view of spatial orientation Eliška was able of independent movement within the interior of the school, she was able to find her spot, she established orientation points, and for orientation she used compensational means, especially support of sense of feel. In orientation within macrospace she was able to use very efficiently her remaining sense of light. In the beginning of her preschool period she was not using security postures, it was possible to see her walking with hands stretched forward - in this context the technique of trailing was explained. She was not afraid of open space, in a known environment - surroundings of school and house - she moves around safely and very naturally. Basic orientation in microspace was on a very good level (orientation "up, down, next to" searching of identical pairs of shapes, she has automatic algorithm of procedures). She was able to count and name shapes. Verbal memory was very well developed. She was able to memorize even more complex poems. When working she was patient, very ambitious with effort to finish each task, failure was not demotivating for her, and she is opened to advices from people around her. In output situation she was able to concentrate, still she got tired rather fast. Eliška was able to communicate in sentences, she understood and accepted commands, verbal communications was developed, articulation flawless. Phonetic hearing was abnormally developed; she was able to reproduce even a more complex rhythm. Her social maturity also corresponded to her age. A slight delayed prerequisites for learning of Brail writing (orientation in a row of numbers, orientation on a plane). Self serving activities were abnormally developed (with respect to severe sight disability), she was led to independence by her parents (dressing up, taking off, stowing the clothes, eating). She was able to use cutlery when eating, she was eating with a spoon independently - only with initial help, it was necessary to describe the position of food on the plate. In the preschool period she also learned to ride a scooter and a bicycle with a sound leader-voice. During manual activities she showed significant patience (e.g. during stringing of beads). Handling was an interesting activity for her - for example distinguishing of coins. Among favorite games was playing with a radio controlled car.

Eliška met basic specialization milestones for given stages, she was improving in social skills, she was very independent, and the psychologist of SPC evaluated overall development very positively. Cooperation of family and school was praised and fruitful.

Advisory body suggested postponing of school attendance - in the postponed year the social pedagogy work was focused on development of requisites for learning of point writing, systematic development of spatial orientation and independent movement, development of lesser and major compensation factors and other specific skills for persons with sight disability. Before entering the elementary school Eliška was able to learn nearly all letters of Brail alphabet, she was able to work very efficiently and in focus. Her sister Tereza was also postponed on elementary school - the parents in principle do not consider varying forms of education. In accord with the wish of parents SPC was preparing conditions for integration to elementary school, cooperation was established with the headmaster of given school, necessary assessments were prepared and material and technical conditions for integration were ensured (aids, textbooks, assistant of the teacher etc.).

Currently Eliška attends for her integration first class of elementary school in her place of residence: It is a class with a smaller number of pupils, her sister Tereza attends the same class. The relations within the class are functioning. The class does not seclude Eliška. Eliška is in intentions of school work very diligent, patient and hard working. Unfortunately, her self reliance is not sufficiently supported (nor by her mother nor by the teacher assistant, nor by the headmaster of the school – for all parties only the fact that she can handle the tempo of the class is important). In stressful situation - in a situation she cannot handle, she is hardheadedly trying to succeed, she can't handle her activeness.

During the entire learning time an assistant of teacher is present in the class. The teacher assistant is not, as special pedagogue puts it, necessary to be present during all classes, in this context in Eliška's case she shall strive for greater independence during classes (organizing part - storing of aids, texts etc. ensures the assistant). The working place is suitably adjusted for Eliška's specific needs (especially sufficient storing space for aids and Brail prints). Eliška uses equal textbooks to her class only in Brail version. She is classified by mark in all subjects, she takes part in all activities of the class and school, in her free time she attends art activity and plays a flute, both ensured by elementary school. Eliška has very good requisites for school work, she is concentrated, she gets oriented in the classes, she works in equal pace as intact schoolmates. One of current tendencies is refusing the touch support - the reason is the attempt for similarity to the group of intact schoolmates. Eliška not only wants to do equal things, she wants to do them in an equal manner, and she strives to blend as best as possible with the rest of the class. In task situation she is not able to react adequately, the touch support is necessary –

this gets her into intensely stressful situation which she demonstrates in panicking.

From the point of view of reading and writing technique of Brail writing she has correct finger distribution and reading technique (she uses both her hands). She checks each individual step. She has slight difficulties in left-right orientation. In mathematics she achieves excellent results; in general she is one of the best in her class.

Equally, her performance in fundaments of civic and natural science is excellent: Eliška´s imagination and work with opinion is positively evaluated. In education she can work independently, in PE she is active, she is herself interested in physical activities, and she has learned exactly the movement paradigms. Stress is put on relaxation exercises and health fitness exercises towards prevention of wrong position of upper body which is manifested especially during sitting and working at a desk. Eliška is evaluated very positively by pedagogues; her approach to school work is highly priced as well as her independence during classes.

In self-serving Eliška aims for maximum independence, orientation in the school environment is secure and safe. Eliška is communicative, direct, she is not afraid to make contact. Acceptance of her disability cannot be judged yet, however, Eliška is very interested in sight disability of others in her coeval group of sight disabled.

Eliška is very content at school, according to her mother she got adapted without problems. Her parents want Eliška to get involved in out of school activities - Eliška started to attend elementary art school (playing flute with a pedagogue with sight disability). Her parents also try to develop her sporting potential - running, swimming, skiing. Special pedagogue finds cooperation with her parents very good.

Currently the situation of Eliška, from cooperation with the family, school, through individual prerequisites as far as contact with the coeval group and fulfillment of socializing tasks of given period, can be evaluated in all aspects as trouble less and positively progressing. In the future it is necessary to support identification with the group of people with sight disability, development of compensational mechanisms and specific competences of individuals with sight disability towards achieving of maximum possible development.

References

Bashour, M. and coll. (2008). Retinopathy of Prematurity: Follow-up. *eMedicine*. (cit. 26. 2. 2009). To be found at WWW: <http://emedicine.medscape.com/article/1225022-followup>.

Dickason, E. J., Silverman, B. L., Schult, M. O. (eds.) (1994). *Maternal-infant nursing care.* 2nd edition. St. Louis: Mosby-Year Book. ISBN 0-8016-7408-5.

Fendrychová, J., Borek, I. and coll. (2007) *Intenzivní péče o novorozence.* 1st edition. Brno: Národní centrum ošetřovatelství a nelékařských zdravotnických oborů. ISBN 978-80-7013-447-4.

Fuchs, V., Zoban, P. and coll. (2001). *Vybrané kapitoly z perinatologie.* 1st edition. Praha: Karolinum. ISBN 80-246-0114-1.

Hendl, J. *Kvalitativní výzkum v pedagogice.* (quote. 14. 5. 2010). To be found at WWW: <www.kpg.zcu.cz/capv/HTML/5/5.pdf>.

Kebza, V., Šolcová, I. (2004). *Komunikace a stres.* 1st edition. Prague: State health institute, ISBN 80-7071-246-5.

Koukola, B., Mareš, J. (2007). *Psychologie zdraví a kvalita života.* Brno: MSD. ISBN 978-80-7392-009-8.

Koukola, B., Mareš, J. (2007). *Psychologie zdraví a kvalita života.* Brno: MSD, ISBN 978-80-7392-009-8.

Kuchynka, P. and coll. (2007). *Oční lékařství.* 1st edition. Prague: Grada, ISBN 978-80-247-1163-8.

Larsson, E. K. and coll. (2007). A Population-based Study on the Visual Outcome in 10-year-old Preterm and Full-term Children. *Arch Ophthalmol*, vol. 123, n. 6, p. 825-832. (cit. 1. 3. 2009). To be found at WWW: http://archopht.ama-assn.org/cgi/content/full/123/6/825?axtoshow=&HITS=10&hits=10&RESULTFORMAT=&fulltext=Health-Related+Quality+of+Life+at+Age+10+Years+in+Very+Low-Birth-Weight+Children+With+and+Without+Threshold+Retinopathy+of+Prematurity&searchid=1&FIRSTINDEX=10&resourcetype=HWCIT.

Leifer, G. (2004). *Úvod do porodnického a pediatrického ošetřovatelství.* 1st edition. Praha: Grada Publishing. ISBN 80-247-0668-7.

Mareš, J. and coll. (2006). *Kvalita života u dětí a dospívajících I.* Brno: MSD, ISBN 80-86633-65-9.

Odehnal, M., Filouš, A. (1998). Retinopatie předčasně narozených dětí. *Česká a slovenská oftalmologie*, vol. 54, pp. 56-64. ISSN 1211-9059.

Rozsíval, P. (2007). *Trendy soudobé oftalmologie.* 1st edition. Praha: Galén. ISBN 978-80-7262-470-6.

Rozsíval, P. and coll. (2005). *Trendy soudobé oftalmologie*. 1st edition. Praha: Galén. ISBN 80-7262-326-5.

Roztočil, A. and coll. (2008). *Moderní porodnictví.* 1st edition. Praha: Grada Publishing. ISBN 978-80-247-1941-2.

Růžičková, V. (2006*). Integrace zrakově postiženého žáka do základní školy.* Olomouc: VUP, ISBN 80-244-1540-2.

Řehulková, O., Řehulka, E., Blatný, M., Mareš, J. et al. (2008). *Kvalita života v souvislostech zdraví a nemocí.* Brno: MSD, ISBN 978-80-7392-073-9.

Salajka, F. (2006). *Hodnocení kvality života u nemocných s bronchiální obstrukcí.* 1st edition Prague: Grada, ISBN 80-247-1306-3.

Schalock, R. L. (2004) The concept of quality of life: What we know and do not know. *Journal of Intellectual Disability Research*, 48, part 3, p. 203-216. (quote. 6. 2. 2010). To be found at WWW:<http://www3. interscience.wiley.com/journal/118795463/issue>.

Silva, L. S., Oliveira, F., Ferreira, L., Pereira, M. (2005). Low vision quality of life assessment: Psychometric validation of Portuguese version of NEI-VFQ 25. *Science Direct*, 1282, s. 729-731. (quote. 18. 5. 2010). To be found at WWW: <http://www.sciencedirect.com/ science?_ob=Article URL>.

Spencer, R. (2006). Long-term visual outcomes in extremely low-birth-weight children (an american ophthalmological society thesis). *Trans Am Ophthalmol Soc*, n. 104, p. 493–516. (cit. 15. 3. 2009). To be found at WWW: <http://www.pubmedcentral.nih.gov/articlerender.fcgi?artid=1809911&tool=pmcentrez>.

Spilker, B. (ed.) (1990). *Quality of Life Assessments in Clinical Trials.* New York: Raven Press Ltd, ISBN 0881675903.

Štembera, Z. (2004). *Historie české perinatologie.* Praha: Maxdorf. ISBN 80-7345-021-6.

Vaďurová, H. (2006). *Sociální aspekty kvality života v onkologii.* 1st edition. Brno: MSD. ISBN 80-86633-60-8.

Vaďurová, H., Mühlpachr, P. (2005). *Kvalita života: teoretická a metodologická východiska.* 1st edition Brno: Masaryk´s University, ISBN 80-210-3754-7.

Zobanová, A. (2005). Dlouhodobé sledování zraku u dětí nejen po retinopatii nedonošených (ROP). *Neonatologické listy*, vol. 11, n. 1, p. 12. ISSN 1211-1600.

In: Retinopathy of Prematurity (ROP)
Editor: Elmira Aguilar

ISBN: 978-1-63482-644-0

Chapter 3

Fractal and Multifractal Analysis of Two Dimensional Images of the Retinopathy of Prematurity: Morphologic Parameters and Classification

Nebojša T. Milošević[1,2*], Nemanja Rajković[1,2] and Herbert F. Jelinek[3]

[1]Department of Biophysics, School of Medicine, University of Belgrade, Serbia

[2]Laboratory for Image Analysis in Medicine, Institute of Biophysics, School of Medicine, University of Belgrade, Serbia

[3]Centre for Research in Complex Systems and School of Community Health, Charles Sturt University, Australia

* Corresponding author: Nebojša T. Milošević, Department of Biophysics, Medical faculty, University of Belgrade, KCS-Institute of biophysics, p. 22, 11102 Belgrade, Serbia. E-mail: mtn@med.bg.ac.rs; nebojsa.milosevic@mfub.bg.ac.rs.

Abstract

Retinopathy of prematurity is a disease caused by abnormal vessel regression of the retinal vasculature that affects premature infants with low birth weights. This paper explores the possibility of applying the concept of fractal analysis to images of retinal blood vessels for morphometric analysis and classification. More than 100 neonates were screening with RetCam 3 device by the experienced ophthalmologist who chose 101 suitable images and set them into three groups, according to the presence of the ROP and the stage of ROP development. Black and white binary images were carried out by box dimension quantifying the space-filling, shape and tortuosity of retinal blood vessels. Accordingly, grey-scale images were investigated by the lacunar and multifractal analysis, which quantifies heterogeneity and multifractal spectra, respectively. The results indicate that the gestational age of premature births did not influence the box dimension, homogeneity and multifractal spectra. The blood vessels in the retinae with severe retinopathy of prematurity are more heterogeneous, complex and have a higher degree of vessel aberration than those vessels with infants without retinopathy. Multifractal analysis, however, did show significant differences between only between those two stages of the retinopathy. We have demonstrated that objective parameters for morphometric analysis and classifying of retinopathy can be found by applying the fractal and multifractal analyses. The next step in developing might be to establish a clinical standard based on fractal and multifractal measures. Another application could be the development of software that can be implemented in standard ophthalmologic imaging.

Keywords: blood vessel, Box dimension, Fractal, Human retina, Lacunarity, Image processing, Multifractal analysis, Retinal vasculature

1. Introduction

Various human blood vessel disorders are associated with obliteration of preexisting blood vessels. Microvessel rarefaction often takes place in the hypertensive lung, in the myocardium of patients with chronic renal failure, and in the elderly [1]. Equally, a failure to eliminate transient embryonic vasculature destined for regression may also lead to disease, as exemplified by persistent hyperplastic primary vitreous, a common congenital developmental anomaly of the eye in which hyaloid vessels fail to regress [2]. A striking example of a disease caused by abnormal vessel regression is retinopathy of prematurity (ROP). The appearance of new blood vessels associated to the development of the retina is an important diagnostic indicator to detect and diagnose vascular and non-vascular pathology either associated with the retina or with other disease [3].

This study explores the possibility of applying the concept of fractal and multifractal analysis to images of blood vessels in the human retina with no-severe and severe ROP in order quantify area and shape of vessels distribution, tortuosity of the vessels, along with heterogeneity of vessel distribution across the retina and their multifractal spectra. Secondary goal was to discriminate two groups of ROP, particularly if fractal parameters were able to diminish ROP1 and ROP2 stage within group of no-severe ROP. In addition, this study explores whether the space-filling and heterogeneity parameters quantified the same or different properties of retinal images with respect to different stages of ROP.

2. Patients, Image Acquisition and Image Preparation

Ocular fundus photography was performed as a part of ROP screening in all infants who had been hospitalized at the Institute for Neonatology (Belgrade, Serbia) during the period of May 2013 to June 2014. The screening criteria included neonates with a gestational age between 32 and 40 weeks or those weighing less than 3000 grams. During the screening examination, the RetCam3 (Clarity Medical Systems, CA, USA), equipped with 130° lens, was used to obtain color images of the retina of both eyes. Pupillary dilation was achieved with two cycles of 0.5% cyclopentolate and 2.5% phenylephrine at 30 minute intervals of instillation. RetCam 3 images were taken by the ophthalmologist-specialist in order to obtain clearly focused images of all parts of the ocular fundus. The images were stored on the RetCam3 computer hard drive. On the basis of ocular findings, 64 infants were identified with good retinal images from a cohort of 135 neonates, and included in this study.

After reviewing the quality of the 128 images, the ophthalmologist-specialist chose 101 suitable images and set them into three groups, according to the presence of the ROP and the stage of ROP development [4]: 19 patients (35 images) with normal diagnosis, i.e. the "Control group," 20 patients (31 images) in "no-severe ROP" group (among them, ROP1 stage had 14 patients-

19 images and ROP2 stage had 6 patients-12 images) and 25 patients (35 images) in "severe ROP" (higher than stage 3 or more). The characteristics recorded for each infant in this study are presented in Table 1.

Table 1. The number of patients, images, interval of gestation and body weight within investigated neonates, with two stages of ROP

Group	Patients	Images	Gestation (week)	Weight (g)
Control	19	35	32-40	750-3000
no-severe ROP	20	31	34-40	900-2000
ROP1 stage	*14*	*19*	*34-38*	*800-1500*
ROP2 stage	*6*	*12*	*34-40*	*800-2000*
severe ROP	25	35	32-40	760-2800

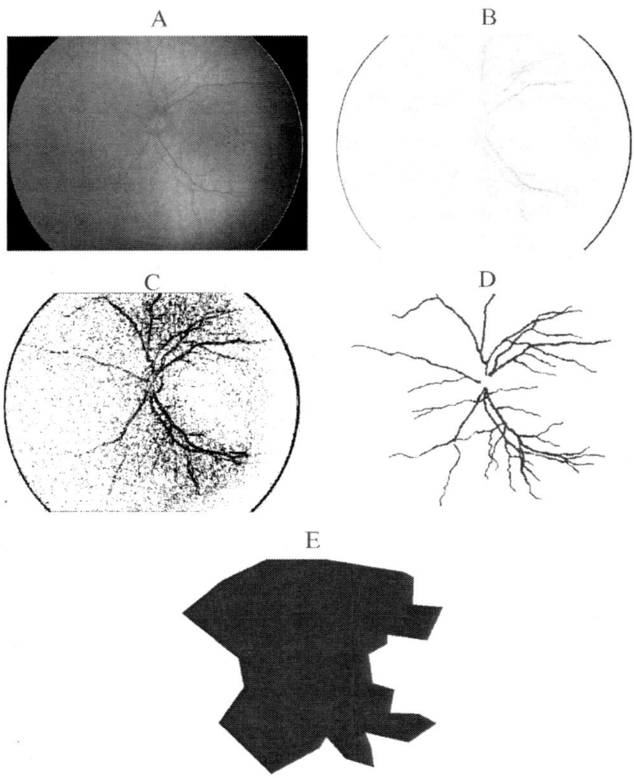

Figure 1. (A-C) From halftone to binary image, (D) final black and white image, after specialist removed all unnecessary objects and edited previous image file, and (E) polygon outline created from previous image.

Each RGB image was imported in software for image analysis, in this case, in Adobe Photoshop CS 5 – Demo version (www.adobe.com/support/downloads).

Figure 1A to 1D presents how a binary (black and white) image of the retina was created using subroutines of previous software: 'Image → Mode → Grayscale' (Figure 1A), than 'Filter → Stylize → Find Edges' (Figure 1B), than 'Image → Adjustment → Threshold (level 240)' (Figure 1C) and finally 'Image → Mode → Binary' (Figure 1D). Before last command, all remaining artifacts (Figure 1C) were digitally removed by the ophthalmologist-specialist, manually editing the file and deleting inadequate objects on the image. At the end, a polygon outline of the each image (Figure 1E), which encompass the tips of the retinal blood vessels within the image [5], was created and saved for further analysis (with the same resolution as image in Figure 1D).

3. Fractal Analysis

Although standard quantitative methods in science are based on classical Euclidean geometry [6], fractal geometry is developed as a new geometry of nature [7]. Generally, the *topological dimension* (D_T) of an object (in space) is defined as the minimum number of coordinates needed to specify a position of any point within it. Early work showed that the most common biological patterns were characterized by fractal geometry [8]. Up to now the concepts of fractal geometry is being used in diverse research areas [7, 8] and is proving to be an increasingly useful tool. In fractal analysis, type of quantitative analysis derived from fractal geometry [9], there are two basic methods to measuring the fractal dimension of objects in a plane: the first and most commonly used is a *length-related method*, while the second method is a *mass-related method* [7]. Most popular method of fractal analysis, and frequently used, is the box-counting method [9]. This section will present how the box-counting method estimate four parameters, applied on two dimensional images of ROP.

3.1. Box-count Dimension

Mathematically, the calculation of the box-counting dimension is easy to apply. The lower and upper box-dimensions of a subset $F \subset R^n$ are respectively defined by

$$\underline{\dim}_B(F) = \underline{\lim}_{\delta \to 0} \frac{\log N_\delta(F)}{-\log \delta}, \quad \overline{\dim}_B(F) = \overline{\lim}_{\delta \to 0} \frac{\log N_\delta(F)}{-\log \delta} \tag{1}$$

and if lower and upper values are equal then the common value is referred to as the box-counting dimension of F and is denoted by

$$\dim_B(F) = \lim_{\delta \to 0} \frac{\log N_\delta(F)}{-\log \delta} \tag{2}$$

where $N_\delta(F)$ can be the smallest number of closed balls of radius δ that cover F, the smallest number of cubes of side δ that cover F, the number of δ-mesh cubes that intersect F, the smallest number of sets of diameter at most δ that cover F or the largest number of disjoint balls of radius δ with centers in F [10].

The box-counting method, applied on 2D digitized images, covers the image with a grid of square cells (with cell size r), where for binary images the cell size is expressed as the number of pixels. The number of squares $N(r)$ needed to cover the image is given by a power law

$$N(r) = \text{const} \cdot r^{-D_B}, \tag{3}$$

where D_B is the box dimension, obtained as an absolute value of the slope of the log-log relationship between $N(r)$ and r [11].

It has been reported previously [8] that the box-counting method applied on binary images (or, black and white images) of neurons depends on image display. While the box dimension of binary-outline images of neurons defines the irregularity in the shape of the image [12], the same parameter for binary-skeletonized images summarizes the degree of dendrite aberrations from straight lines [5]. In addition, the box dimension of the binary images of neurons represents a robust technique for estimating how the extent of the neuron deviates from the extent of the geometric figure, according to resolution [12].

Figure 2A illustrates how the box-counting method can estimate the extent of a filled square, which center is in same position as the image of the retina. When the box-counting method was applied on the black image of the square (Figure 2A, gray square), the log $N(r)$-log r relationship can be fitted with "perfect" straight line (i.e. $R^2 = 1$) and the absolute value of such a slope gives $D_B = 2$, which represents fractal dimension of the area (Figure 2B). Figure 2C demonstrates how a polygon outline of the vessels was created by joining each vessel ending which is not cut by other vessels by a line [11].

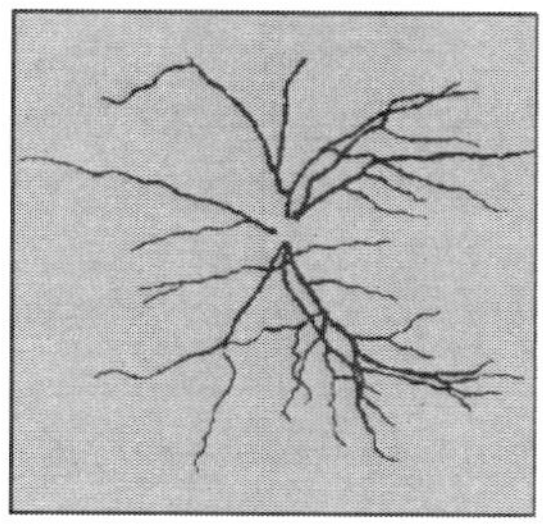

A

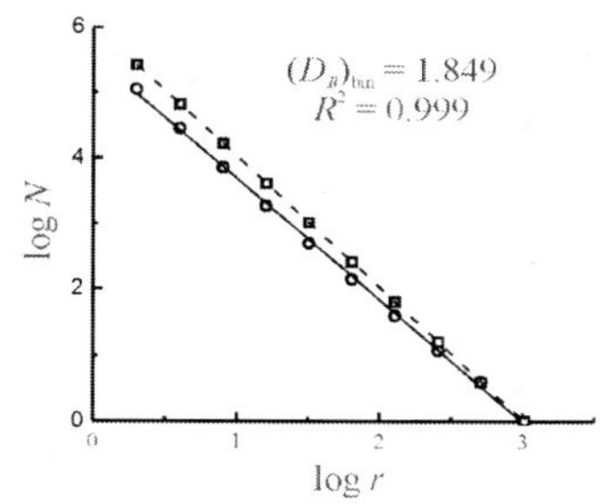

B

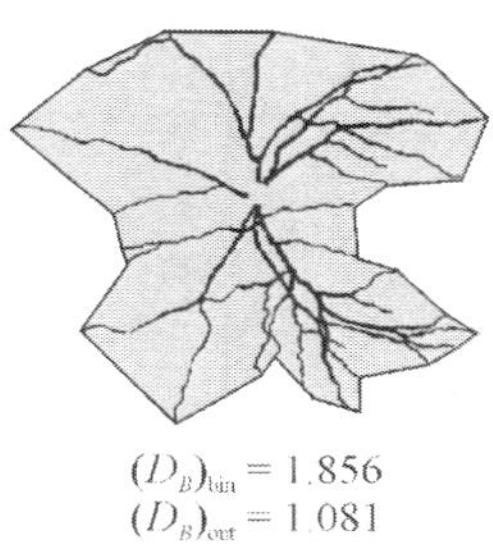

C

Figure 2. A) The binary image of the retina encompassed by the square, B) Log-log plot between number of squares (N) and square size (r) for the binary image (circles and line) encompassed by the square (squares and dashed line). D_B is the absolute value of the slope of the regression line and R^2 is the corresponding determination coefficient. C) A polygon outline (gray color, different shade from first image) of the vessels. The values of the $(D_B)_{\text{bin}}$ and $(D_B)_{\text{out}}$ are in lower part of picture.

3.2. The Lacunarity

In fractal analysis, lacunarity (usually denoted as Λ or λ) is more generally a measure of 'visual texture' in images [13, 14]. It has been defined as the degree of *gappiness*, *inhomogeneity*, and *translational and rotational invariance* in an image [7]. Low lacunarity implies homogeneity, equated to having mostly similarly sized gaps and little rotational variance, while high lacunarity implies heterogeneity or having many differently sized gaps and notable rotational variance [7]. Figure 3 demonstrates an example of a low and high value of lacunarity on the halftone images.

A B

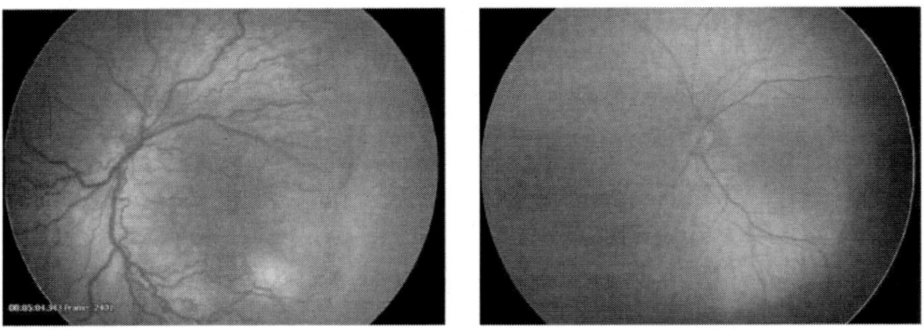

$\Lambda = 0.559$ $\Lambda = 0.372$

Figure 3. An example of high (A) and low (B) lacunarity obtained on the halftone RetCam images.

In box counting, lacunarity is determined from the probability distribution for pixels, sometimes called the mass distribution. The distribution is determined from the number of pixels per box as a function of box size or scale (ε). Lacunarity at a particular ε (λ_ε) is calculated as

$$\lambda_\varepsilon = (CV)^2 = \left(\frac{\sigma}{\mu}\right)^2 \tag{4}$$

where (CV) is the coefficient of variation, σ is the standard deviation and μ the mean of the pixels per box at ε [7]. To arrive at a single number [13], the values for λ_ε can be summarized as the mean λ for the total number of calibers (E)

$$\bar{\lambda} = \frac{\sum \lambda_\varepsilon}{E}. \tag{5}$$

3.3. Fractal Parameters of the Vessel Morphology

All parameters were calculated either in Image J or in the FracLac plugin of Image J [15], which was set to the box-counting procedure. The space-filling property of the vessel distribution across the retina was evaluated with $(D_B)_{\text{bin}}$ on the corresponding black and white image (Figure 1D). The vessel irregularity and complexity was investigated after the binary images of the retinal blood vessels (Figure 1D) were skeletonized and $(D_B)_{\text{skel}}$ was obtained. The shape of the vessel distribution was estimated with $(D_B)_{\text{out}}$, which was calculated from the polygon outline of the each image encompassing the tips of the retinal blood vessels within the image [5] (Figure 1E). The box sizes were taken from 2^1 to 2^k pixel, where k is the value for which $N = 1$. As for our material, the box size spanned from 2 to 1024 pixels or from 2 to 2048 pixels, depending on the image size. Finally, the lacunarity (Λ) was obtained on the halftone (or gray-scale) retinal images (Figure 1A).

In order to test whether gestational age is correlated with the current morphological features determined from the box counting method, the values of $(D_B)_{\text{bin}}$, $(D_B)_{\text{out}}$, $(D_B)_{\text{skel}}$ and Λ were statistically evaluated (Table 2). Gestational age spanned from 32 to 40 week (Table 1), with the number of infants, in each group (no-severe ROP and severe ROP), varying from 31 to 35 images and tabulated t value is equal for the both groups (2.042, $p < 0.05$). Thus, calculated t values for parameters shown in Table 2 were smaller than the tabulated value.

Table 2. The values of the determination coefficient (R^2) and calculated t value for the binary, skeletonized and outline box dimension, along with the lacunarity in two groups of the ROP

Parameters	No-severe ROP		Severe ROP		p
	R^2	t_{cal}	R^2	t_{cal}	
$(D_B)_{\text{bin}}$	0.058	1.422	0.018	0.845	> 0.05
$(D_B)_{\text{skel}}$	0.012	0.633	0.016	0.796	
$(D_B)_{\text{out}}$	0.075	1.636	0.026	1.020	
Λ	0.018	0.778	0.083	1.879	

Table 3 shows the central tendency and dispersion measure of the box dimensions ($(D_B)_{bin}$, $(D_B)_{skel}$, and $(D_B)_{out}$) and lacunarity (Λ) for all three groups, along between ROP1 and ROP2 within no-severe ROP group. As can be seen from this table, infants with severe ROP have high means of $(D_B)_{out}$ and $(D_B)_{skel}$, than other two groups, while the opposite is found for $(D_B)_{out}$ and Λ in no-severe ROP and control group, respectively. Since the sample sizes (i.e. images) between groups are unequal (Table 1), the Scheffé *post hoc* test [16] for all possible pairwise comparisons was applied.

The calculated *t*-values were significantly different to the tabulated value indicating a significant difference: between control and other two groups for $(D_B)_{bin}$ ($p < 0.01$ and $p < 0.05$), between control and severe ROP for $(D_B)_{out}$ ($p < 0.05$), between all pairs for $(D_B)_{skel}$ ($p < 0.001$) and between control and no-severe ROP for Λ ($p < 0.05$). Finally, only for $(D_B)_{skel}$, Kolmogorov Smirnov-testing [16] confirmed normal distributions and *t*-testing yielded significant ($p < 0.05$) difference between ROP1 and ROP2 subgroup of no-severe ROP group (Table 3).

Table 3. The values of four parameters ($(D_B)_{bin}$, $(D_B)_{out}$, $(D_B)_{skel}$ and Λ) for normal group (A) and two stages of the ROP: no-severe (B) and severe ROP(C). Also four parameters are shown for ROP1 and ROP2 within no-severe ROP group. Each value is shown as the mean ± standard error, while within ROP1 and ROP2 values are shown as the median ± range

Group	$(D_B)_{bin}$	$(D_B)_{out}$	$(D_B)_{skel}$	Λ
A	1.813 ± 0.002 **[B]	1.073 ± 0.004 *[C]	1.107 ± 0.004	0.47 ± 0.01
B	1.822 ± 0.002 *[C]	1.078 ± 0.004	1.151 ± 0.007 ***[A]	0.44 ± 0.01 *[A]
C	1.818 ± 0.002	1.084 ± 0.004	1.220 ± 0.004 ***[A,B]	0.46 ± 0.01
ROP1	1.824 ± 0.017	1.071 ± 0.052	1.088 ± 0.056 *[ROP2]	0.42 ± 0.15
ROP2	1.823 ± 0.024	1.073 ± 0.046	1.176 ± 0.063	0.45 ± 0.13

* - $p < 0.05$, ** - $p < 0.01$, *** - $p < 0.001$.

To investigate the possible interaction between $(D_B)_{bin}$ and Λ, data was plotted for the two groups of the ROP (Figure 4). When the regression lines were observed, $(D_B)_{bin}$ decreased when Λ increased, particularly for "no ROP" group (Figure 4A). But when the Spearman-Rank correlation test [16] was applied, between $(D_B)_{bin}$ and Λ no significant negative correlation was found

(Figure 4) indicating that there was no correlation between $(D_B)_{\text{bin}}$ and Λ for both ROP groups.

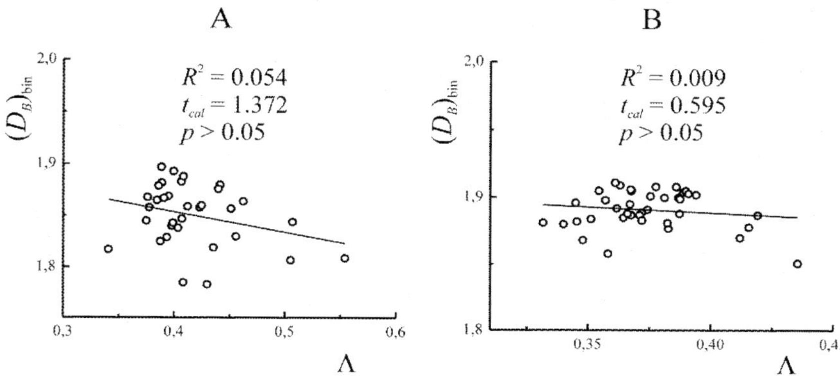

Figure 4. Plots of $(D_B)_{\text{bin}}$ versus Λ for no-severe ROP(A) and severe ROP (B) groups of infants. Data were fitted with a straight line (regression). The coefficient of determination (R^2), calculated t value and level of confidence (p) were inscribed in the upper part of each plot.

4. Multifractal Analysis

Multifractals are special types of fractal which scale with multiple scaling rules. As we look in some pattern on picture it is not easy to determine whether a pattern is multifactal or not, so the use of mutifractal analysis is required. Main goal of this analysis is to detect property of *multi* in scaling [13, 17, 18]. The essential calculations for doing multifractal analysis using box-counting technique is present here.

The standard box-count lays series of grids, with decreasing box size, over the image and assess how the size of the box affects the number of boxes of foreground pixels within the image. In contrast to previous approach, multifractal analysis with box-counting technique estimate distribution of pixel values in a digital image. That is, the series of grids gather information about the distribution of pixel values (we know it as "mass distribution") over the image, and became the basis for a series of calculations which explore the multiple scaling rules.

As we said before, to resolve whether is pattern multifractal or not, we need to create multifractal spectra from the pattern. Easiest way is to create spectra from the series of generalized dimensions calculated over some arbitrary range. If the range is denoted with Q then generalized dimension is presented with symbol D_Q. To find D_Q, the mean probability distribution at scale (ε) is exaggerated by being raised to the arbitrary exponent (i.e. the Q), and then compared again to how the exaggeration varies with scale ε. Therefore, D_Q basically addresses how mass varies with ε in an image, or how mass behaves when an image is resolved into a series of ε-sized pieces and distorted by Q. Thus, D_Q is defined by equation

$$D_Q = \frac{\lim\limits_{\varepsilon \to 0}\left(\frac{\ln I_{Q,\varepsilon}}{\ln \varepsilon^{-1}}\right)}{1-Q} \tag{5}$$

where $I_{Q,\varepsilon}$ is distribution of pixels (inspected at some ε), defined by

$$I_{Q,\varepsilon} = \sum_{1}^{N_\varepsilon} P_{i,\varepsilon}^{Q} \tag{6}$$

where N_ε represents number of boxes containing pixels and $P_{i,\varepsilon}{}^{Q}$ is the sum of all probabilities at each box (or scale).

An alternative multifractal measure is the $f(\alpha)$ multifractal spectrum (DeBartolo et al. 2000). According to the method of [19] this multifractal spectrum is calculated using

$$\mu_{i(Q,\varepsilon)} = \frac{P_{i(Q,\varepsilon)}^{Q}}{\sum\limits_{i=1}^{N_\tau} P_{i(Q,\varepsilon)}^{Q}} \tag{7}$$

to find

$$\alpha_{(Q)} = \frac{\sum\limits_{i=1}^{N_\tau} \mu_{i(Q,\varepsilon)} \cdot \ln P_{i(Q,\varepsilon)}}{\ln \varepsilon} \tag{8}$$

and finally,

$$f(\alpha(Q)) = \frac{\sum_{i=1}^{N_\tau} \mu_{i(Q,\varepsilon)} \cdot \ln \mu_{i(Q,\varepsilon)}}{\ln \varepsilon}. \tag{9}$$

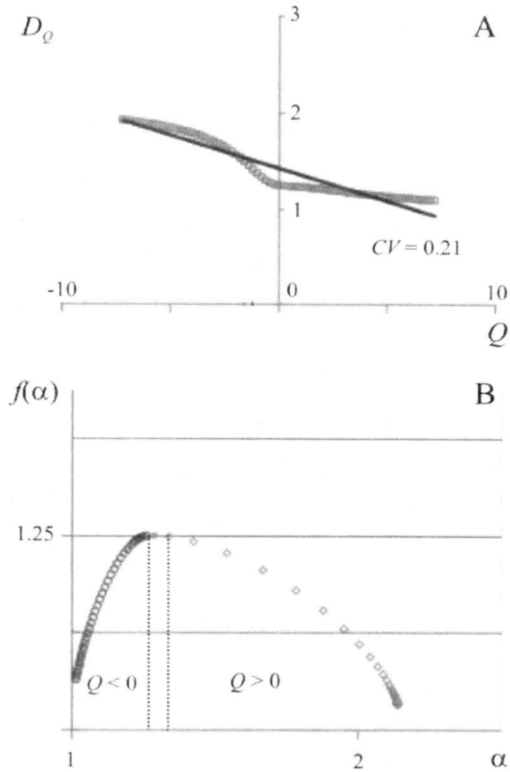

Figure 5. Relations between D_Q and Q (A), and $f(\alpha)$ and α (B) in multifractal spectra for the Henon map (http://imagej.nih.gov/ij/plugins/fgm/).

Simply speaking, multifractal spectra are graphs showing how a pattern behaves if amplified in certain ways. If a pattern scales uniformly (i.e. as in monofractal) distorting the probability distribution reveals little change. But if a pattern scales non-uniformly (as happens with multifractals), distinct mathematical views emerge as the multifractal spectra. For monofractals, the function D_Q is usually either essentially unchanging or decreasing around zero point, with low dispersion or low value of the coefficient of variation (*CV*, defined as the ratio of the standard deviation and the mean of the regression line). But for multifractals, D_Q typically sigmoidally decreases around zero, with high dispersion (high *CV*).

In contrast to D_Q, the function $f(\alpha)$, show a different pattern. While the convergence is obvious for monofractals, especially for positive Q, for multifractals the $f(\alpha)$ rises and falls with increase of Q, showing maximum (i.e. the capacity dimension or global fractal dimension) for $Q = 0$. Figure 3 demonstrates for the Henon map (http://imagej.nih.gov/ij/plugins/fgm/index.html) theoretical fractal with multifractal properties, relationships D_Q vs. Q and $f(\alpha)$ vs. α.

Figure 6 shows multifractal spectra for normal group (squares), group with no-severe ROP (triangles) and group with severe ROP (diamonds). For all Qs (smaller or higher from zero) severe ROP group had higher data than no-severe group and normal group, respectively. The multifractal spectra indicated that there was some variation in the degree of multifractal scaling in all groups, although for Qs between (-1, 1) fractal dimension looks statistically similar. Based on ANOVA for the scales of Q applied, there were significant differences between all groups for $Q \leq -2$, and between normal and severe ROP for $Q \geq 3$. This analysis was not capable to discriminate no-severe group on ROP1 (19 images) and ROP2 (12 images) subgroup.

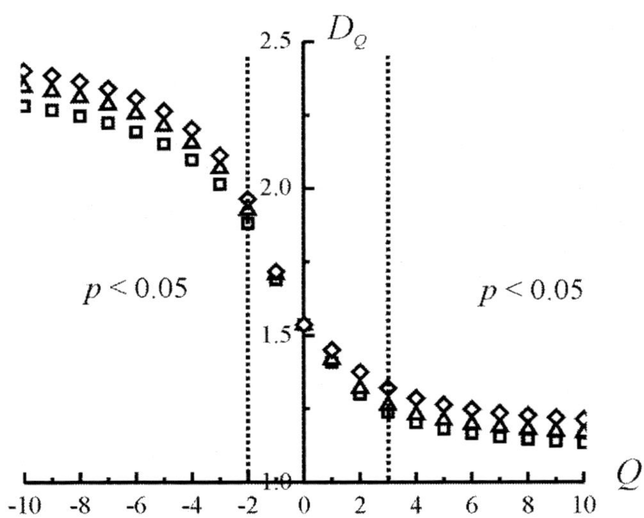

Figure 6. Multifractal spectra (D_Q vs Q) for normal (squares), no-severe ROP (triangles) and severe ROP group (diamonds). Dashed lines and symbols (*- $p < 0.05$ and **- $p < 0.01$) indicate intervals with significant difference.

5. Discussion

5.1. Image Analysis of the Retinal Blood Vessel

Analysis of the retinal vessel structure is of immense interest for the investigation of diseases that involve structural or functional changes within the retinal vasculature. Changes to the retinal vasculature, such as hemorrhages, angiogenesis, vessel tortuosity, blockages and diameter are important indicators of diabetic retinopathy, ROP and cardiovascular risk [20-22].

Optic fundus assessment is an important diagnostic indicator for detection and diagnosing of non-vascular and vascular pathology [20]. The assessment of retinal blood vessels from optic fundus photography requires segmentation of the vessels from the background, so that suitable feature extraction and processing may be performed [23]. Segmentation methods vary depending on the imaging modality and application domain [22]. There is a growing body of literature on the segmentation of blood vessels from retinal images that provide comparisons between methods and methods for segmentation of images [15]. In contrast to these studies, this study promotes a different method of acquisition of the optic fundus images using RetCam 3. The default resolution of the image (100 dpi), absence of the ruler and the fact that arteries, veins and various artifacts were linked on the image, was main reasons why expert (ophthalmologist) analyzed and segmented original images.

Vessels and arteries have many observable features [Hoover], including diameter, color, tortuosity (relative curvature) and opacity (reflectivity). Following segmentation, a vascular network can be defined in terms of bifurcation angles and junction exponents at branching points as well as tortuosity, curvature and opacity [15].

In the present study we applied four morphometric parameters, which describe the space distribution, shape, irregularity and homogeneity of vessels across the retinae, along with multifractal analysis and proved the hypothesis that the morphology of retinal vessels in premature birth infants was not influenced by gestational age when infants are assessed between 32 and 40 weeks (Table 2).

5.2. Fractal and Multifractal Analysis of Retinal Blood Vessels

Fractal analysis is a set of mathematical techniques used to quantify complex structures [12, 24]. Namely, the fractal dimension of a structure expresses numerically the degree of geometrical complexity of that structure [8, 12]. The global fractal dimension of the retinal vasculature has been studied for some time and shown to be influenced by diabetes and other diseases affecting the arteries, veins or both [25-27].

To the best of our knowledge, box-counting analysis of the retinal blood vessels in the ROP has not yet been extensively investigated [28], contrary to other methods where the fractal analysis of retinal blood vessels has been studied extensively [15, 20, 29-31].

This study therefore explored the possibility of applying a standard box-counting analysis to the images of blood vessels in the human retinae. Generally, the outline and skeletonized box dimensions of images in infants with diagnosed severe ROP are higher, than the box dimensions of same images in infants without ROP or no-severe ROP (Table 3). The opposite conclusion can be drawn for binary box dimension and lacunarity, where "no-severe" and control group have highest binary box dimension and lacunarity, respectively. This result proved the hypothesis that the retinal blood vessel distribution is more homogenous and vessels are less irregular in patients with normal diagnosis (i.e. the control group).

Several research groups have demonstrated that the normal retinal vasculature has fractal-like properties with a global dimension generally falling between 1.60 and 1.88 [25, 27, 32] for retinal cameras using 60% visual angle. Our results do confirm previous findings, although we used a different method for estimating global dimension than previous research. An important novel finding was that our results indicate that the increase in lacunarity was not followed by a decrease or increase in binary box dimension (Figure 4) or *vice versa*. Thus, the binary box dimension and lacunarity estimate different properties on the image of retinal vessels: space-filling and inhomogeneity and provide useful tools for the assessment of ROP.

Multifractal properties is relevant to patterns in which a spectrum of fractal dimensions can be identified rather than a single global dimension. Multifractal systems are common in nature and our analysis indicates that the type of retinal images discussed in this paper also has these characteristics and may provide additional information to the clinician with reference to the scale of investigation. By using these methods we show, that it is possible to find significant differences between images with "no-severe" and "severe" ROP.

Although we found one potential limitation in that there was no statistically significant difference between two subgroups of "no-severe" ROP multifractal analysis, however, did show significant differences between "severe" ROP and normal diagnosis.

5.3. Morphology and Classification of ROP2

ROP is a blindness-causing neovascularizing disease that affects premature birth infants treated with high concentrations of oxygen [1] and may ultimately lead to retinal detachment and vision loss [4]. ROP develops in two distinct stages [1]: first, the hyperoxic insult leads to obliteration of immature retinal vessels; the second phase is an adverse compensatory neovascularization response, mediated by ischemia-induced vascular endothelial growth factor (VEGF). The trend toward early treatment of high-risk patients emphasizes the importance for early detection of ROP, particularly the "severe" stage of the ROP. This stage occurs among the smallest of low-birth-weight neonates and progresses rapidly into more severe forms of the disease, which may not follow the classic stages of typical ROP [33].

The system used for describing the findings of active ROP is entitled *The International Classification of Retinopathy of Prematurity* (ICROP), which uses a number of parameters to describe the disease [33]. They are location of the disease into zones, the circumferential extent of the disease based on the clock hours, the severity of the disease and the presence or absence of "Plus Disease." Each aspect of the classification has a technical definition, all of them were used for the major clinical trials [33].

First and second stage of ROP do not lead to blindness, although they can progress to the more severe stages. In terms of blindness, they can be summarized into "no-severe" group of ROP. As *threshold disease* is defined as disease that has a 50% likelihood of progressing to retinal detachment, this form is considered to be present when stage 3 ROP is present in either first or second zone, with at least 5 continuous or 8 total clock hours of disease, and the presence of *plus* disease [34]. Progression to partial or total retinal detachment, will result in substantial or total loss of vision for the infant. In our study, such images (or patients) were classified into "severe" ROP group. Although two groups were discriminated from normal retinal vasculature due to the tortuosity of vessels (Table 3), analysis of the vessel distribution and inhomogeneity have showed that "no-severe" group was different from normal patients (control group), while group of "severe" ROP was different from control only in the shape of distribution (Table 3). Between "no-severe" and "severe" group difference was found in vessel distribution and tortuosity. Finally, between ROP1 and ROP2 subgroup of "no-severe" group (first and second stage of ROP) difference was found in vessel tortuosity only. It is most likely that number of images (Table 1 – statistically small sample) is responsible for such result in stage classification.

Conclusion

The results shown in this study are encouraging, particularly as the box dimension (or the fractal dimension in general) has proven to be a useful parameter for quantifying images with ROP and their classification. The current study can be considered as a good start for further investigation, particularly when additional stages of retinopathy, with more patients (or images) are included. Such analysis of the blood vessels can lead to a more reliable interpretation of retinal disease, disease progression and treatment effectiveness.

Compared to other approaches, the proposed methods are fast, easy and reliable. The next step in developing this technology is to establish a clinical standard based on fractal measures. Involvement of a larger number of images could help to reinforce this effort. Another application could be the development of software that yields a specific prognosis, e.g. using fractal dimensions to predict various stages of ROP identified in multifractal spectra.

Acknowledgment

Authors want to thank Prof. Ana Oros (Department of Ophthalmology, School of Medicine University of Novi Sad, Serbia) for images of retinal blood vessels in premature infants and in analysis and segmentation of original images.

References

[1] E. Keshet, Preventing pathological regression of blood vessels, *J. Clin. Invest.* 112 (2003) 27-29.

[2] J. N. Upalakalin, I. Hemo, C. Dehio, E. Keshet and L.E. Benjamin, Survival mechanisms during vascular remodeling, *Cold Spring Harbor Symp. Quant. Biol.* 67, (2002) 181-187.

[3] D. Hughes, E. Martinez-Perez, A. S. Jabbar, A. Hassan, N. W. Witt, P. D. Mistry, N. Chapman, A. V. Stanton, G. Beevers, R. Pedrinelli, K. H. Parker and S. A. Thom, Quantification of topological changes in retinal vascular architecture in essential and malignant hypertension. *J. Hypertens.* 24 (2006) 889–894.

[4] Cryotherapy for Retinopathy of Prematurity Cooperative Group, Multicenter trial for cryotherapy for retinopathy of prematurity Ophthalmological outcomes at 10 years, *Arc. Ophthal.* 119 (2001) 1110-1118.

[5] D. Ristanović, N. T. Milošević, B. D. Stefanović, D. L. Marić and K. Rajković, Morphology and classification of large neurons in the adult human dentate nucleus: A qualitative and quantitative analysis of 2D images. *Neurosci. Res.* 67 (2010) 1-7.

[6] B. B. Mandelbrot, *The Fractal Geometry of Nature*, WH Freeman and Co., New York, USA (1983).

[7] T. G. Smith Jr, G.D. Lange and W.B. Marks, Fractal methods and results in cellular morphology: dimensions, lacunarity and multifractals, *J. Neurosci. Methods* 69, (1996) 123–136.

[8] E. Fernández and H. F. Jelinek, Use of fractal theory in neuroscience: methods, advantages, and potential problems, *Methods* 24 (2001) 309–321.

[9] N. T. Milošević, B. Krstonosić, G. N. Elston and N. Rajković N, Box-count analysis of two dimensional images: methodology, analysis and classification. In: Dumitrache I, Magda Florea A, Pop F (eds.) *Proceedings of 19th International Conference on Control Systems and Computer Science, Vol. 2: Interdisciplinary approaches in fractal analysis IAFA 2013*, The Institute of Electrical and Electronics Engineers, Los Alamitos, CA, USA, (2013) 306-312.

[10] K. Falconer, *Fractal geometry: Mathematical foundation and applications, second edition*, John Wiley & Sons, England (2003).

[11] N. T. Milošević, D. Ristanović, H. F. Jelinek, and K. Rajković, Quantitative analysis of dendritic morphology of the alpha and delta retinal ganglion cells in the rat: a cell classification study. *J. Theor. Biol.* 259 (2009) 142-150.

[12] N. T. Milošević, D. Ristanović and K. Rajković, Mathematical Model of Box-Counting Analysis in the Human Dentate Nucleus during Development. In: G. Banaszak, P. Waliszewski (eds.) *Fractals and Complexity*, Poland: Cracow, (2012) 40-46.

[13] Karperien, H.F. Jelinek and N. T. Milošević, Multifractals: a review with an application in neuroscience. *Proceedings CSCS-18, Vol. 2: Interdisciplinary approaches in fractal analysis IAFA 2011*, R. Dobrescu (ed.), Editura Politehnica Press, Bucharest, Romania, (2011) 888-893.

[14] S. Talu, C. Vladutiu, L.A. Popescu, C.A. Lupascu, S.C. Vesa and S.D. Talu, Fractal and lacunarity analysis of human retinal vessel arborisation in normal and amblyopic eyes. *Hum. Vet. Medicine* 5, (2013) 45-51.

[15] Karperien, H. F. Jelinek, J. J. G. Leandro, J. V. B. Soares, R. M. Cesar Jr and A. Luckie, Automated detection of proliferative retinopathy in clinical practice. *Clin. Ophtalmol.* 2 (2008) 109-122.

[16] R. H. Riffenburgh, Statistics in medicine. San Diego-London: Academic press, (1999).

[17] T. Vicsek, *Fractal Growth Phenomena*, World Scientific, Singapore, (1992).

[18] F. Jestczemski, M. Sernetz, Multifractal approach to inhomogeneous fractals. *Physica A* 223 (1996) 275-282.

[19] Chhabra, R. V. Jensen, Direct determination of the f(a) singularity spectrum. *The American Physical Society* 62 (1989) 1327-1330.

[20] R. Nekovei, and Y. Sun, Back-propagation network and its configuration for blood vessel detection in angiograms. *IEEE Trans. Neur. Net.* 6 (1995) 64-72.

[21] N. Patton, T. M. Aslam, T. MacGillivray, I. J. Deary, B. Dhillon, R. H. Eikelboom, K. Yogesan and I. J. Constable, Retinal image analysis: concepts, applications and potential. *Prog. Retin. Eye Res.* 25 (2006) 99-127.

[22] Fenster and B. Chiu, Evaluation of segmentation algorithms for medical imaging. *IEEE Eng. Med. Biol.* 7 (2005) 7186-7189.

[23] S. Talu, The influence of the retinal blood vessels segmentation algorithm on the monofractal dimension. *Oftalmologia* 56 (2012) 73-83.

[24] N. T. Milošević, M. Olujić, A. Oros and H.F. Jelinek, Retinopathy of Prematurity: Fractal Analysis of Images in Different Stages of the

Disease. In: I. Dumitrache (ed). *Advances In Intelligent Control Systems and Computers Science*. Springer-Verlag, Berlin-Heidelberg, (2013) p. 91.

[25] Daxer, Fractals and retinal vessels, *Lancet* 339 (1992) p. 618.

[26] G. Liew, J. J. Wang, P. Mitchell and T. Y. Wong, Retinal vascular imaging: a new tool in microvascular disease research, *Circ. Cardiovasc. Imag.* 1 (2008) 156-161.

[27] F. Family, B. R. Masters, and D. E. Platt, Fractal pattern formation in human retinal vessels. *Physica D* 38 (1989) 98-103.

[28] R. M. Cesar Jr and H. F. Jelinek, Segmentation of retinal fundus vasculature in nonmydriatic camera images using wavelets. In: Suri, J.S., Laxminarayan, S. (Eds.) *Angiography and Plaque Imaging*, CRC Press, Boca Raton, Florida, (2003) 193-224.

[29] J. V. B. Soares, J. J. G. Leandro, R. M. Cesar Jr, H. F. Jelinek and M. J. Cree, Retinal vessel segmentation using the 2-D Gabor wavelet and supervised classification. *IEEE Trans. Med. Imag.* 25 (2006) 1214-1222.

[30] X. W. Gao, A. Bharath, A. Stanton, A. Hughes, N. Chapman and S. Thom, Quantification and characterisation of arteries in retinal images, *Comp. Meth. Prog. Biomed.* 63 (2000) 133-146.

[31] J. Staal, M. D. Abramoff, M. Niemeijer, M. A. Viergever, and B. van Ginneken, Ridgebased vessel segmentation in color images of the retina, *IEEE Trans. Med. Imaging* 23 (2004) 501–509.

[32] G. Landini, P.I. Murray and G.P. Misson, Local connected fractal dimensions and lacunarity analyses of 60 degrees fluorescein angiograms. *Invest. Ophthalmol. Vis. Sci.* 36, (1995) 2749-2755.

[33] Committee for the Classification of Retinopathy of Prematurity, The International Classification of Retinopathy of Prematurity revisited. *Arch. Ophthalmol.* 123 (2005) 991-999.

[34] D. L. Phelps, Retinopathy of Prematurity: history, classification and pathophysiology. *NeoReviews* 2(2001) 153-166.

In: Retinopathy of Prematurity (ROP)
Editor: Elmira Aguilar
ISBN: 978-1-63482-644-0

Chapter 4

Management of Retinopathy of Prematurity: Past and Future

Gordon Shing Kin Yau**, *Jacky Wai Yip Lee, Benjamin Chung Yin Chu and Victor Tak Yau Tam
Department of Ophthalmology, Caritas Medical Centre, Hong Kong SAR, China

Abstract

Retinopathy of prematurity (ROP) is a vaso-proliferative disease targeting the developing retina particularly in those with low birth weight and preterm gestation.

Despite significant improvements in screening guidelines and treatment modalities, ROP is still the leading cause of reversible paediatric blindness worldwide. The 1984 Classification of Retinopathy of Prematurity and the 1988 Cyrotherapy for ROP (CRYO-ROP) study made screening for ROP imperative and subsequently improved the visual prognosis of this condition. The aim of screening is to detect infants with ROP and to deliver treatment in a timely manner to prevent irreversible visual loss. With advancements in the field of neonatology, smaller and sicker infants are surviving and therefore ROP continues to be a growing medical and public concern.

* Corresponding author: Gordon Shing Kin YAU, E-mail: skyau0303@gmail.com.

Differences in ethnicity and socioeconomic status influence the prevalence, risks, outcome, and management of ROP. In this chapter, the incidences, risk factors, screening guidelines, and treatment trends will be reviewed and the characteristics in various preterm subtypes (extremely low birth weight, extremely preterm, multiple pregnancies, and co-twins) will also be highlighted with reference to their risks in ROP development.

1. Introduction

Retinopathy of prematurity (ROP) was first recognized in 1942 when Terry published a description of histological findings in advanced cicatricial ROP [1]. As more cases were reported, it became evident that the disease was confined to premature infants and retrospective studies showed that the disease was rarily recognized before 1942. Terry (1945) [2] and later Owens et al. (1948) [3] showed that the retinopathy developed in infants who had a normal fundal examination at birth, demonstrating that the disease developed in postnatal life. ROP subsequently became the leading cause of blindness in children in the developed countries like the United States followed by a similar epidemic in Europe during the 1950's [4, 5].

Campbell suggested that the onset of ROP was closely related to the introduction of oxygen therapy during the neonatal period supporting the concept of a toxic effect of oxygen on the immature retinal vasculature [6]. However many other factors play a role in the pathogenesis of as described later by Lucey et al. [7] and Ben Sira et al. [8].

Nowadays, it is well known that ROP is a retinal vaso-proliferative disease affecting low birth weight (BW) pre-term neonates especially in those having stormy postnatal periods and exposure to high ambient oxygen concentrations. The retina is unique in that there are no blood vessels until the fourth month of gestation at which time vascular complexes emanating from the hyaloids vessels at the optic disc grow towards the periphery. These vessels reach the nasal periphery after 8 months of gestation, and they do not reach the temporal periphery until about 1 month after delivery. This incompletely vascularized temporal retina is particularly susceptible to oxygen damage (even in normal atmospheric oxygen).

It was evidenced by in vitro studies that the avascular zone of the retina releases vascular endothelial growth factors (VEGF), leading to the development of abnormal fibro-vascularization [9, 10]. These abnormal fibro-vascular tissues will form various ridges and traction and exert pulling forces onto the edge of the immature retina. Eventually the retina bleeds, exudates form and eventually detaches in the final stages. Thus, ROP was previously known as retro-lental fibroplasia.

Despite having improved classification guidelines and treatment modalities, ROP is still the leading cause of reversible paediatric blindness especially in developed nations [4, 5]. The 1984 Classification of ROP [11] and the 1988 CRYO-ROP study [12] made screening for ROP imperative and subsequently improved the visual prognosis of this condition. The aim of screening is to detect infants with ROP who require treatment and to facilitate an earlier window for treatment. Prompt and appropriate treatment can prevent blindness for the infant, medical intervention for ROP is vital on both an individual level and for the society on a whole. With advancements in paediatric resuscitation skills and modern medical equipment, smaller and lighter infants are surviving and therefore ROP presents a growing medical and public concern [13-15].

2. Epidemiology

Two epidemics of ROP occurred in the past 70 years. The first occurred between the 1940-50's, resulting from the introduction of the neonatal incubator that supplied supplementary oxygen therapy [6, 16]. High hyperoxemia causes premature obliteration of retinal vessels in premature infants.

This realization led to the change in policy of reducing supplementary oxygen for premature infants [17-20]. Despite more vigilant monitoring of supplementary oxygen therapy use in preterm infants, the second epidemic of ROP occurred in between the1970-80's due to the increasing survival rate of extreme preterm infants following medical advancements in developed countries [21]. With these advances in neonatology and improvements in survival rate of extremely preterm and low birth weight infants in the past decades, mandatory ROP screening protocols were established in the majority of developed countries like United kingdom (UK), United States (USA), and Australia. It has been postulated that there may soon be a third epidemic of ROP in these countries due to the survival of weaker and smaller babies [22-24].

The incidence of the ROP varies among different research studies and populations. In the CRYO-ROP study conducted from 23 centres in the united states with recruitment of 9751 infants, 65.8% of infants developed ROP while 6% required treatment to halt disease progression [25]. In the Early Treatment of ROP study (ET-ROP) study, 68% of infants developed ROP [26]. These two large multicentre studies had similar incidences because they shared the same inclusion criteria. (birth weight < 1251 grams). However, on most occasions, screening guidelines vary among different countries making it difficult to directly compare ROP incidences [27].

3. International Classifications

The International Classification of ROP (ICROP) was published in 3 parts, in 1984, 1987further, and again modified in 2005 incorporating standardised clinical images as reference [28-30]. It was revised as a consensus from a group of international experts in ROP in hope to improve understanding of this disorder and to facilitate clinical trials [30].

3.1. Disease Course

The grading of active ROP can be determined according to (a) location and extent, (b) severity/staging of the disease:

(a) Location is determined according to 3 zones centred on the optic disc and extent is denoted in clock hours (Figure 1).

Zone I	The area of a circle centred at fovea with radius twice of distance between optic disc and fovea
Zone II	A circle is drawn with the optic disc as the centre and disc to nasal ora serrata as the radius. The area between zone I and this boundary constitutes zone II
Zone III	The temporal arc of retina remaining beyond the radius of zone II is zone III
Extent	The extent is denoted by the clock hours of retinal involvement in that particular zone.

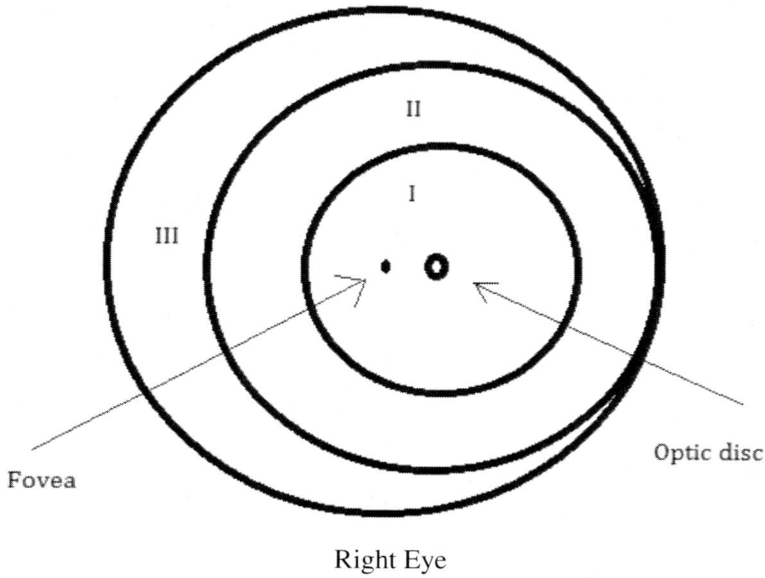

Figure 1. The retina is divided into 3 zones centered on the optic disc.

(b)

Table 1. Severity/staging of disease

Severity	Description	Characteristics
Stage 1	Demarcation Line	• The first pathognomonic sign of active ROP • A thin, tortuous, grey white line that is seen at the edge of vessels, dividing the vascular from the avascular retina
Stage 2	Ridge	• If the ROP progresses, the demarcation line develops into a ridge of tissue which extends out from the plane of the retina
Stage 3	Extra-retinal fibrovascular proliferation	• As the disease progresses, the ridge becomes pink as a result of the development of fibrovascular proliferation along the surface of the retina and into the vitreous

Table 1. (Continued)

Severity	Description	Characteristics
Stage 4a	Subtotal retinal detachment not involving the macula	• A tractional retinal detachment which starts in the extreme periphery and then spread centrally
Stage 4b	Subtotal retinal detachment involving the macula	• With this stage onwards prognosis for vision becomes poor
Stage 5	Total retinal detachment (funnel-shaped)	• The funnel is divided into anterior and posterior parts allowing 4subdivisions, depending upon whether the funnel is open or narrow in both parts
Plus Disease		• Dilatation and tortuosity of 2 vessels in the posterior quadrants, or • Vitreous haze, or • Pre-retinal vitreous haemorrhage, or • Engorgement of the iris vessels and pupillary rigidity
Pre-plus disease	Pre-plus disease early in the course of ROP is strongly associated with the development of severe ROP that require laser treatment	• Vascular abnormalities of the posterior pole that are insufficient for the diagnosis of plus disease but that demonstrate more arteriolar tortuosity and more venular dilatation than normal
Aggressive Posterior ROP (APROP) (previously termed "Rush Disease")	This is rapidly progressive ROP in the posterior pole, usually seen in extremely ill babies	• The disease may bypass the early stages and progress to stage 5 rapidly. • Prominence of plus disease with ill defined stages. • It needs prompt treatment(< 48 hours).

Table 2. Screening Criteria of UK and USA with reference usingn the most updated guideline[33, 36]

UK-ROP 2008 guideline	USA ROP 2013 guideline
All babies less than 32 weeks gestational age (GA) (up to 31 weeks and 6 days) or less than 1501g birth weight should be screened for ROP. One criterion to be met for inclusion.	Infants with a BW ≤ 1500 g or gestational age ≤ 30week and 6 day
All babies less than 31 weeks gestational age (up to 30 weeks and 6 days) or less than 1251 grams BW must be screened for ROP. One criterion to be met for inclusion.	Any premature babies with BW between 1.5 – 2.0 kg are considered to have higher risk of ROP if judged by neonatologists to have an unstable clinical course in terms of cardio-respiratory support

Table 3. Timing of the first ROP screening

Gestational Age (Weeks)	Timing of the first ROP screening			
	Postnatal Weeks		*Postmenstrual Weeks*	
	UK	*USA*	*UK*	*USA*
22	8	9	30	31
23	7	8	30	31
24	6	7	30	31
25	5	6	30	31
26	4	5	30	31
27	4	4	31	31
28	4	4	32	32
29	4	4	33	33
30	4	4	34	34
31	4	4	35	35
32 or older	4	4	postnatal 4 weeks	

Babies < 32 weeks gestational age or BW < 1501 grams should have their first ROP screening examination prior to discharge. The ophthalmic findings at the first eye examination and subsequent examinations will dictate the minimum follow-up frequencies required to detect and provide timely intervention for those with rapid progression or high risks.

4. Screening Guidelines in the UK and USA

Screening Criteria and Protocols

Timely screening and treatment can substantially reduceunfavourable visual outcomes [12]. Subsequently, guidelines for screening time, follow up intervals, and treatment criteria of ROP have been drawn up by different nations. The 2 most commonly used guidelines are from the UK and USA.

Table 4. Frequencies of ROP screening

Minimum Subsequent Screening Examinations Frequencies should be:	
UK ROP 2008 guideline	**USA ROP 2013 guideline**
Weekly	**1-Week or Less**
• The vessels end in zone I or posterior zone II; or • There is any plus or pre-plus disease; or • There is any stage 3 disease in any zone	• Immature vascularization: zone I— • no ROP • Immature retina extends into posterior zone II, near the boundary of zone I • Stage 1 or 2 ROP: zone I • Stage 3 ROP: zone II • The presence or suspected presence of aggressive posterior ROP
	1- to 2-Weeks
	• Immature vascularization; posterior zone II • Stage 2 ROP: zone II • Unequivocally regressing ROP: zone • I
Minimum Subsequent Screening Examinations Frequencies should be:	
UK ROP 2008 guideline	**USA ROP 2013 guideline**
Weekly	**1-Week or Less**
Every 2 weeks:	2-Weekly
• In all other circumstances until the criteria for termination have been reached	• Stage 1 ROP: zone II • Immature vascularization: zone II (no ROP) • Unequivocally regressing ROP: zone II
	2- to 3-Weekly
	• Stage 1 or 2 ROP: zone III • Regressing ROP: zone III

The UK-ROP screening guideline was published by the British Association of Perinatal Medicine and then by the College of

Ophthalmologists in 1990 and was revised in 1995 with the most updated guidelines issued in 2008 [31-33].

The USA guideline was issued by the American Academy of Pediatrics, American Academy of Ophthalmology and American Association for Pediatric Ophthalmology and Strabismus in 1997 [34]. It was revised in2001 and 2006 with the most updated recommendation issued in 2013 [35, 36].

Although there are minor differences between these 2 well established screening recommendations, it is still valuable to compare and contrast these 2 guidelines.

Any delays in ROP screening may cause missing of the limited window of opportunity for treatment, leading to devastating outcomes. The decision to postpone a screening examination is made on clinical grounds and it should be a joint decision between the ophthalmologists and neonatologists with carefully balancing the risks of delaying diagnosis of sight threatening ROP versus the systemic co-morbidities induced by the stress of screening babies during stormy postnatal periods. If a deferment is decided, a repeated examination should be rescheduled within 1 week [33].

Table 5. Termination of ROP screening

Termination of ROP Screening	
UK ROP 2008 guideline	**USA ROP 2013 guideline**
• In babies without ROP, there is minimal risk of developing sight threatening ROP when vascularisation has extended into zone III and ROP screening may be stopped at this juncture wich usually occurs after 36 weeks postmenstrual age	• Zone III retinal vascularization attained without previous zone I or II ROP
• In the presence of ROP, screening for progressive active disease may be discontinued when any of the following characteristics of regression are seen on at least 2 successive examinations: • Lack of increase in severity • Partial resolution progressing towards complete resolution • Change in colour in the ridge from salmon pink to white • Transgression of vessels through the demarcation line • Formation of scar tissue	• Full retinal vascularization in close proximity to the ora serrate for 360° • (This criterion should be used for all cases treated for ROP solely with bevacizumab) • Postmenstrual age of 50 weeks and no pre-threshold disease (defined as stage 3 ROP in zone II, any ROP in zone I) or no further worsening ROP is detected • Regression of ROP

5. Risk Factors for Rop and Type 1 Rop Development

Extremely low BW (< 1,000 grams) and extreme preterm (GA < 28 weeks) infants are well known to be associated with higher risk of development of ROP and Type I ROP (formly termed "threshold ROP") [12, 38-41]. Multiple prenatal, perinatal and postnatal risk factors have been studied to identify their associations with ROP development.

A higher targeted oxygen saturation (SaO_2) has detrimental effect on the lungs and the eyes of preterm infants [42-44]. The reported incidence of Type I ROP in the first Australian Benefits Of Oxygen Saturation Targeting (BOOST) trial reported incidences of 16% in the standard target oxygen-saturation group (SaO_2 91-94%) and 8% for the high oxygen-saturation group. In the BOOST-II study, the incidence was 10.6% in the lower target saturation group and 13.5% in the higher-target group [42, 43].

Studies by Yau et al. in Hong Kong revealed that multiple pregnancies and invasive mechanical ventilation were associated with the development of the more aggressive Type 1 ROP on univariate analysis [45] while the presence of intraventricular hemorrhage, thrombocytopenia was associated with development of any stage of ROP [46].

Several other risk factors has been identified for the development of ROP and more severe forms of ROP including: congenital heart diseases [47]; anemia [48]; inotrope use in the management of postnatal hypotension [49]; use of erythropoietin [50]; vaginal delivery [51]; neonatal sepsis [52]; necrotising enterocolitis; bronchopulmonary dysplasia; and light exposure [53].

6. Treatment Criteria and Therapeutic Modalities

Timely treatment for ROP is imperative in preventing severe visual loss. The CRYO-ROP study in 1980's recommended treatment for threshold disease (presence of stage 3 plus ROP in at least 5 contiguous or 8 cumulative clock hours in zone I or II. The CRYO-ROP study reported a poor visual outcome in 25.7% of eyes treated with cryotherapy versus 47.7% in untreated eyes at 1 year ($P < 0.0001$) and 30.0% versus 51.9% in treated and untreated eyes respectively at 15 years [12, 54, 55].

Later, the multicentre Early treatment-ROP (ETROP) trial compared early treatment of high-risk prethreshold (Table 6) with conventional threshold treatment. The study revealed an overall significant benefit from early treatment in eyes with high-risk prethreshold disease that tend of have less unfavourable visual acuities and structural outcomes. The study further divided ROP severity into Type I and Type II Prethreshold ROP (Table 6) [56, 57].

Treatment of APROP should be within the 48 hours, while other forms of ROP requiring treatment should generally be conducted within 72 hours to minimize the risk of retinal detachment. Follow-up is recommended in 3 to 7 days after treatment to ensure that there is no need for additional treatment in areas where ablative treatment was incomplete and follow-up should be continued at weekly intervals at minimum, for signs of decreasing ROP activity and regression.

Treatment options included cryotherapy, trans-pupillary indirect laser (argon or diode) ablative therapy [58]. When there is stage 4 or 5 disease (retinal detachment), vitreo-retinal surgery is required to salvage the eyes. Despite recent advances in the vitero-retinal surgical techniques, the anatomical and the visual outcome of stage 4 and 5 disease are always poor [59].

Table 6. Definition of Prethreshold ROP used in the ETROP trial

Term	Definition
Prethreshold	• Zone I, any stage ROP less than threshold • Zone II, Stage 2 with plus disease • Zone II, Stage 3 without plus disease • Zone II, Stage 3 with plus disease, but less than the criteria for threshold disease

Table 7. Definition of Type I and Type II Prethreshold disease from the ETROP trial

Type I Prethreshold ROP	Zone I, any Stage ROP with plus disease Zone I, Stage 3 with or without plus Zone II, Stage 2 or 3 ROP with plus disease
Type II Prethreshold ROP	Zone I, Stage 1 or 2 ROP without plus disease Zone II, Stage 3 ROP without plus disease

The following ophthalmic criteria are therefore recommended to identify babies requiring ROP treatment.

Treatment for ROP should be undertaken if any of the following indications are reached:

- Zone I, any stage of ROP with plus disease,
- Zone I, Stage 3 without plus disease,
- Zone II, Stage 3 with plus disease.
- Babies with aggressive posterior ROP (APROP)

Treatment for ROP should be seriously considered if the following indication is reached:

- Zone II, Stage 2 with plus disease

In recent years, the efficacy of intravitreal bevacizumab for Stage 3+ Retinopathy of Prematurity (BEAT-ROP) study revealed the intravitreal bevacizumab monotherapy compared to conventional laser ablative therapy, was superior in Zone I Stage 3 plus disease with the benefit of progressive vascularization at the peripheral avascular zone [60]. However, there are still several issues related to the intravitreal bevacizumab injection that need to resolved before it can be launched for wide spread clinical use for ROP:

a) The safety, dosage, and timing of injection
b) Bevacizumab is currently not approved by the Food and Drug Administration in USA for intravitreal injection
c) The longer post-treatment follow-up required as compared to laser therapy to detected the late recurrence of ROP

8. Future Developments in Rop Screening

8.1. Tele-medicine

With advances in the neonatal intensive care, more survivals in premature deliveries will be expected, leading to the growing need for ROP care worldwide. Specialists or experts in ROP staging may frequently not be available in every single hospital. Thus, wide-field digital imaging systems can help to capture and centralize ROP screening by remote ROP experts. This new technology has potential to improve accessibility, quality, and cost of ROP management [61].

8.2. Should We Screening Fewer Babies?

The administrative and financial burden of ROP screening on the healthcare system will continue to increase in the future. ROP screening is not only costly but also uncomfortable for the neonate and thus, should really be reserved for those at risk. ROP screening guidelines will need to undergo regular updates and modifications that are specific to the local population in order to provide an cost effective, evidence-based screening protocol yet maintaining an efficient practice without over-screening [62]. Several methods have been discussed to reduce the number of the infants being screening while not missing any case of severe ROP. Base on a retrospective case series by Mathew et al. they found that all severe ROP (Stage 3 and threshold ROP) were babies with BW < 1000 grams and GA < 28 weeks. Thus, they recommended a refinement the screening inclusion criteria to reduce the number of babies been screened [63]. Later, Yang et al. used a multivariate risk-based screening protocol to increase the efficiency of ROP screening for infants with BW between 401-1250 grams without an apparent loss of effectiveness, thus reducing the mean number of eye examinations per infant (P = 0.0051) [64]. Van Sorge et al. from the Netherlands recommended that ROP screening may be reduced by factoring risk factor to each infant's postnatal course including BW, GA, artificial ventilation, sepsis, necrotizing enterocolitis, postnatal glucocorticoids use and cardiotonica [65]. Morerecently, Ying G et al. formulated the ROP prediction model using predictive factors that could identify high-risk infants who require more intensive examinations a while reducing examinations for those with lower risks [66].

Conculsion

With the technological advances in neonatal care, smaller, lighter, and more premature infants are surviving. ROP will likely continue to be an important healthcare issue in the years to come. While BW and GA are 2 of the most established risk factors, studies have reported a variety of prenatal, perinatal, and postnatal risk factors that may influence the development and severity of ROP. Since the incidence and characteristics of ROP can vary among populations of difference race and socioeconimical status, ROP screening guidelines must incorporate the disease characteristics that are unique to the population being screened. Screening can be enhanced via the inclusion of predictive factors for ROP or the involvement of experts via telemedicine when there is insufficient expertise. Prompt treatment and close follow-up are essential in visual preservation for ROP requiring treatment as late stage disease often has poor prognosis despite treatment. While photocoagulative therapy has been the predominate modality of treatment, future studies involving the long-term outcome of anti-vascular endothelial growth factors may change the treatment practice and prognosis of ROP.

References

[1] Terry, TL. Extreme prematurity and fiboblastic overgrowth of persistent vascular sheath behind each crystalline lens. *Am J Ophthalmol.,* 1942, 25, 203-4.

[2] Terry, TL. Retrolental fibroplasia in premature infants. Further studies on fibrolastic overgrowth of tunica vasculosa lentis. *Arch Ophthalmol.,* 1945, 33, 203-8.

[3] Owens, WC; Owens, EU. Retrolental fibroplasia in premature infants. *Trans Am Acad Ophthalmol Otolaryngol.*, 1948, 53, 18-41.

[4] Steinkuller, PG; Du, L; Gilbert, C; Foster, A; Collins, ML, Coats, DK.Childhood blindness. *J AAPOS*. 1999, 3, 26–32.

[5] Yau, GS; Lee, JW; Tam, VT; Liu, CC; Chu, BC; Yuen, CY. Incidence and risk factors for retinopathy of prematurity in extreme low birth weight Chinese infants. *Int Ophthalmol*. 2014 Jun 5. [Epub ahead of print]. DOI 10.1007/s10792-014-9956-2.

[6] Campbell, K. Intensive oxygen therapy as a possible cause for retrolental fibroplasia. A clinical approach. *Med J Austr.*, 1951, 2, 48-50.

[7] Lucey, JL; Dangman, B. A re-examination of the role of oxygen in retrolental fibroplasia. *Pediatrics*. 1984, 73, 82-96.

[8] Ben, Sira, I; Nissenkorn, I; Kremer, I. Retinopathy of prematurity. *Surv Ophthalmol*, 1988, 33, 1-16.

[9] Sato, T; Kusaka, S; Shimojo, H; Fujikado, T. Vitreous levels of erythropoietin and vascular endothelial growth factor in eyes with retinopathy of prematurity. *Ophthalmology*, 2009, 116, 1599- 603.

[10] Sonmez, K; Drenser, KA; Capone, A, Jr; Trese, MT. Vitreous levels of stromal cell-derived factor 1 and vascular endothelial growth factor in patients with retinopathy of prematurity. *Ophthalmology*. 2008, 115, 1065-1070.

[11] An international classification of retinopathy of prematurity. *Pediatrics*, 1984, 74 (1), 127-33.

[12] Cryotherapy for Retinopathy of Prematurity Cooperative Group. Multicenter trial of cryotherapy for retinopathy of prematurity: preliminary results. *Arch Ophthalmol*. 1988, 106 (4), 471-479.

[13] Gong, A; Anday, E; Boros, S; Bucciarelli, R; Burchfield, D; Zucker, J; Long W. The American Exosurf Neonatal Study Group I (1995) One-year follow-up evaluation of 260 premature infants with respiratory distress syndrome and birth weights of 700 to 1,350 g randomised to two rescue doses of synthetic surfactant or air placebo. *J Pediatr*, 126, S68–S74/

[14] Kennedy, J; Todd, DA; Watts, J; John, E. (1997). Retinopathy of prematurity in infants less than 29 weeks' gestation: 3 1/2 years pre-and postsurfactant. *J Pediatr Ophthalmol Strabismus*., *34*, 289–292.

[15] Termote, J; Schalij-Delfos, NE; Brouwers, HA; Donders, AR; Cats, BP. (2000). New developments in neonatology: less severe retinopathy of prematurity? *J Pediatr Ophthalmol Strabismus*., *37*(3), 142–148.

[16] Saugstad, OD. Is oxygen more toxic than currently believed? *Pediatrics*, 2001, 108, 1203–05.

[17] Michaelson, IC. The mode of development of the vascular system of the retina with some observations on its significance for certain retinal diseases. *Trans Ophthalmol Soc*., 1948, 68, 137–180.

[18] Ashton, N; Ward, B; Serpell, G. Effect of oxygen on developing retinal vessels with particular reference to the problem of retrolental fibroplasia. *Br J Ophthalmol*., 1954, 38, 397–432.

[19] Patz, A; Eastham, A; Higginbotham, DH; Kleh, T. Oxygen studies in retrolental fibroplasia. *Am J Ophthalmol*., 1953, 36, 1511–1522.

[20] Lutty, GA; Chan-Ling, T; Phelps, DL; et al. Proceedings of the Third International Symposium on Retinopathy of Prematurity: an update on ROP from the lab to the nursery (November 2003, Anaheim, California) *Mol Vis*., 2006, 12, 532–580.

[21] Gilbert, C. Retinopathy of prematurity; a global perspective of the epidemics, population of babies at risk and implications for control. *Early Hum Dev.*, 2008, 84, 77-82.

[22] Bouzas, L; Bauer, G; Novali, L, et al. Retinopathy of prematurity in the XXI century in a developing country; an emergency that should be resolved. *Annals de paediatrica.*, 2007, 66, 551-8.

[23] Chen, Y; Li, X. Characteristics of severe retinopathy of prematurity patients in China: a repeat of the first epidemic? *Br J Ophthal.*, 2006, 90, 268-271.

[24] Vikas, Tah; Walid, Sharif; Imran, Yusuf; Marcus, Posner; Louise, Ramskold; Farihah, Tariq; Dev, Mukhey; Zuhair, Sharif. (2014). Retinopathy of Prematurity, *Ophthalmology* - Current Clinical and Research Updates, Associate Prof. Pinakin Davey (Ed.), ISBN: 978-953-51-1721-6, InTech, DOI: 10.5772/58585. Available from: http://www.intechopen. com/books/*ophthalmology*-current-clinical-and-research-updates/retinopathy-of-prematurity

[25] Palmer, EA; Flynn, JT; Hardy, RJ; et al. The cryotherapy for retinopathy cooperative study group. Incidence and early course of ROP. *Ophthalmology.* 1991, 98, 1628-1640.

[26] Good, VW; Hardy, RJ; Dobson, V, et al. Early Treatment for Retinopathy of Prematurity Cooperative Study Group. The incidence and course of retinopathy of prematurity; findings from the early treatment for retinopathy of prematurity study. *Pediatrics.* 2005, 116, 15-23 (http://pediatrics.aappublications.org/cgi/content/full/116/1/15).

[27] Gergely, K; Gerinec, A. Retinopathy of prematurity--epidemics, incidence, prevalence, blindness. *Bratisl Lek Listy.* 2010, 111(9), 514-7.

[28] An international classification of retinopathy of prematurity. *Pediatrics*, 1984, 74 (1), 127-33.

[29] Aaberg; Thomas; et al. "An international classification of retinopathy of prematurity: II. The classification of retinal detachment." Archives of *Ophthalmology*, 105.7 (1987), 906-912.

[30] The International Classification of Retinopathy of Prematurity revisited. The International Committee for the Classification of Retinopathy of Prematurity. *Arch Ophthalmol.*, 2005, 123.

[31] Anonymous. College news: ROP Screening Duty. Quart Bull Coll *Ophthalmol.*, 1990, Autumn, 6.

[32] The report of a Joint Working Party of The Royal College of Ophthalmologists and the British Association of Perinatal Medicine

Retinopathy of prematurity: guidelines for screening and treatment. *Early Hum Dev*, 1996, 46(3), 239-258.

[33] Royal College of Paediatrics and Child Health. Guideline for the screening and treatment of retinopathy of prematurity. http://www.rcpch.ac.uk (Accessed on 2 Nov 2014)

[34] Screening examination of premature infants for retinopathy of prematurity. A joint statement of the American Academy of Pediatrics, the American Association for Pediatric *Ophthalmology* and Strabismus, and the American Academy of *Ophthalmology. Pediatrics.*, 1997 Aug, 100(2 Pt 1), 273.

[35] Section on *Ophthalmology* American Academy of Pediatrics; American Academy of *Ophthalmology*; American Association for Pediatric *Ophthalmology* and Strabismus. Screening examination of premature infants for retinopathy of prematurity. *Pediatrics.* 2006 Feb, 117(2), 572-6.

[36] Fierson WM; American Academy of Pediatrics Section on *Ophthalmology*; American Academy of *Ophthalmology*; American Association for Pediatric *Ophthalmology* and Strabismus; American Association of Certified Orthoptists. Screening examination of premature infants for retinopathy of prematurity. *Pediatrics.* 2013 Jan, 131(1), 189-95. doi:10.1542/peds.2012-2996. Epub 2012 Dec 31.

[37] Hutchinson, AK; Saunders, RA; O'Neil, JW; Lovering, A; Wilson, ME. Timing of initial screening examinations for retinopathy of prematurity. *Arch Ophthalmol.*, 1998, 116(5), 608–612.

[38] Markestad, T; Kaaresen, PI; Rønnestad, A; et al. Norwegian extreme prematurity study group. Early death, morbidity, and need of treatment among extremely premature infants. *Pediatrics.*, 2005, 115, 1289–1298.

[39] Austeng, D; Ka¨llen, KB; Ewald, UW; et al. Incidence of retinopathy of prematurity in infants born before 27 weeks' gestation in Sweden. *Arch Ophthalmol.* 2009, 127, 1315–1319. doi:10.1001/archophthalmol. 2009.244.

[40] Austeng, D; Blennow, M; Ewald, U; et al. Incidence of and risk factors for neonatal morbidity after active perinatal care: extremely preterm infants study in Sweden (EXPRESS). Acta Paediatr. 2010, 99, 978–992. doi:10.1111/j.1651-2227.2010.01846.x.

[41] Brian, A. Darlow; Jolie, L. Hutchinson; David, J. Henderson-Smart; Deborah, A. Donoghue; Judy, M. Simpson; Nicholas, J. Evans; and on behalf of the Australian and New Zealand Neonatal Network. Prenatal Risk Factors for Severe Retinopathy of Prematurity Among Very

Preterm Infants of the Australian and New Zealand Neonatal Network. *Pediatrics*. 2005, 115, 4 990-996, doi:10.1542/peds.2004-1309

[42] Askie, LM; Henderson-Smart, DJ; Irwig, L; Simpson, JM. Oxygen saturationtargets and outcomes in extremely preterm infants. N Engl J Med. 2003, 349, 959–967. doi:10.1056/NEJMoa023080.

[43] The BOOST II United Kingdom, Australia, New Zealand Collaborative Groups. Oxygen saturation and outcomes in preterm infants. N Engl J Med. 2013, 368, 2094–2104. doi:10.1056/NEJMoa1302298.

[44] Supplemental Therapeutic Oxygen for Prethreshold Retinopathy of Prematurity (STOP-ROP), a randomized, controlled trial. I: Primary outcomes. Pediatrics 2000, 105, 295-310.

[45] Yau, GS; Lee, JW; Tam, VT; Liu, CC; Wong, IY. Risk factors for retinopathy of prematurity in extremely preterm Chinese infants. Medicine (Baltimore). 2014 Dec, 93(28), e314. doi:10.1097/ MD.0000000000000314.

[46] Yau, GS; Lee, JW; Tam, VT; Yip, S; Cheng, E; Liu, CC; Chu, BC; Yuen, CY. Differences in risk factors for retinopathy of prematurity development in paired twins: a Chinese population study. *Scientific World Journal.*, 2014, 2014, 212183. doi: 10.1155/2014/212183. Epub 2014 Oct 23.

[47] Polito, A; Piga, S; Cogo, PE; Corchia, C; Carnielli, V; Da Fre`, M; Di Lallo D; Favia, I; Gagliardi, L; Macagno, F; Miniaci, S; Cuttini, M. Increased morbidity and mortality in very preterm/VLBW infants with congenital heart disease. *Intensive Care Med.*, 2013. 39(6), 1104–1112. doi:10.1007/s00134-013-2887-y

[48] Englert, JA; Saunders, RA; Purohit, D; Hulsey, TC; Ebeling, M. The effect of anemia on retinopathy of prematurity in extremely low birth weight infants. *J Perinatol.*, 2001. 21(1), 21–26.

[49] Mizoguchi, MB; Chu, TG; Murphy, FM; et al. Dopamine use is an indicator for the development of threshold retinopathy of prematurity. *Br J Ophthalmol.* 1999, 83, 425–428.

[50] Manzoni, P; Memo, L; Mostert, M; Gallo, E; Guardione, R; Maestri, A; Saia, OS; Opramolla, A; Calabrese, S; Tavella, E; Luparia, M; Farina, D. Use of erythropoietin is associated with threshold retinopathy of prematurity (ROP) in preterm ELBW neonates: a retrospective, cohort study from two large tertiary NICUs in Italy. *Early Hum Dev.*, 2014 Sep, 90 Suppl 2, S29-33. doi: 10.1016/S0378-3782(14)50009-6.

[51] Manzoni, P; Farina, D; Maestri, A; Giovannozzi, C; Leonessa, ML; Arisio, R; Gomirato, G. Mode of delivery and threshold retinopathy of

prematurity in pre-term ELBW neonates. *Acta Paediatr.*, 2007 Feb, 96(2), 221-6.

[52] Manzoni, P; Maestri, A; Leonessa, M; Mostert, M; Farina, D; Gomirato, G. Fungal and bacterial sepsis and threshold ROP in preterm very low birth weight neonates. *J Perinatol.*, 2006 Jan 1, 26(1), 23-30.

[53] Kopylov, U; Sirota, L; Linder, N. Retinopathy of prematurity--risk factors. *Harefuah*. 2002 Dec, 141(12), 1066-9, 1089.

[54] Cryotherapy for Retinopathy of Prematurity Cooperative Group. Multicenter trial of cryotherapy for retinopathy of prematurity. One-year outcome-structure and function. *Arch Ophthalmol,* 1990, 108(10), 1408-1416.

[55] Palmer, EA; Hardy, RJ; Dobson, V; Phelps, DL; Quinn, GE; Summers, CG, et al. Cryotherapy for Retinopathy of Prematurity Cooperative Group. 15-year outcomes following threshold retinopathy of prematurity: final results from the multicenter trial of cryotherapy for retinopathy of prematurity. *Arch Ophthalmol*, 2005, 123(3), 311-318.

[56] Good, WV; Early Treatment for Retinopathy of Prematurity Cooperative Group. Final results of the Early Treatment for Retinopathy of Prematurity (ETROP) randomized trial. *Trans Am Ophthalmol Soc*, 2004, 102, 233-248.

[57] Good, WV; Early Treatment for Retinopathy of Prematurity Cooperative Group. The early treatment for retinopathy of prematurity study (ETROP): Structural findings at 2 years of age. *Br J Ophthalmol*, 2006, 90(11), 1378-1382.

[58] McNamara, J; Tasman, WS; Brown, GC; Vander, JF. Laser photocoagulation for threshold retinopathy of prematurity. In Proc. International Conference on Retinopathy of Prematurity, Chicago IL USA 1993. Eds Shapiro MJ, Biglan AW, Miller MT. Kugler Publications, *Amsterdam*. 1995, 103-7.

[59] Charles, SC. Surgical results for vitrectomy for stage 5 ROP. In Proc. International Conference on Retinopathy of Prematurity, Chicago IL USA 1993. Eds Shapiro MJ, Biglan AW, Miller MT. Kugler Publications, *Amsterdam*, 1995, 181-2.

[60] Mintz-Hittner, HA; Kennedy, KA; Chuang, AZ;, BEAT-ROP, Cooperative, Group. Efficacy of intravitreal bevacizumab for stage 3+ retinopathy of prematurity. *N Engl J Med.*, 2011, 1.364(7), 603–615

[61] Richter, GM; Williams, SL; Starren, J; Flynn, JT; Chiang, MF. Telemedicine for retinopathy of prematurity diagnosis: evaluation and

challenges. *Surv Ophthalmol.*, 2009 Nov-Dec, 54(6), 671-85. doi: 10.1016/j.survophthal.2009.02.020.

[62] Ko, CY; Lee, SY; Chan, WM; Tsang, MK; Tse, RKK; Chow, CB. Should fewer babies be screened for retinopathy of prematurity? *HKJ Ophthalmol.*, 5(1), 21-24.

[63] Mathew, MR; Fern, AI; Hill, R. Retinopathy of prematurity: are we screening too many babies? *Eye (Lond).*, 2002 Sep, 16(5), 538-42.

[64] Yang, MB; Donovan, EF. Risk analysis and an alternative protocol for reduction of screening for retinopathy of prematurity. *JAAPOS*. 2009 Dec, 13(6), 539-45. doi: 10.1016/j.jaapos.2009.10.002.

[65] van Sorge, AJ; Schalij-Delfos, NE; Kerkhoff, FT; van Rijn, LJ; van Hillegersberg, JL; van Liempt, IL; Peer, PG; Simonsz, HJ; Termote, JU. Reduction in screening for retinopathy of prematurity through risk factor adjusted inclusion criteria. *Br J Ophthalmol.*, 2013 Sep, 97(9), 1143-7. doi: 10.1136/bjophthalmol-2013-303123. Epub 2013 Jul 3.

[66] Ying, G; Quinn, GE; Wade, KC; Repka, MX; Baumritter, A; Daniel, E; for the e-ROP Cooperative Group. Predictors for the Development of Referral-Warranted Retinopathy of Prematurity in the Telemedicine Approaches to Evaluating Acute-Phase Retinopathy of Prematurity (e-ROP) Study. *JAMA Ophthalmol.* 2014 Dec 18. doi: 10.1001/jamaophthalmol.2014.5185.

In: Retinopathy of Prematurity (ROP)
Editor: Elmira Aguilar
ISBN: 978-1-63482-644-0

Chapter 5

Indirect Diode Laser Photocoagulation in the Treatment of Retinopathy of Prematurity

Simona Delia Nicoară[1*] and Tudor Cătălin Drugan[2]
[1]"Iuliu Hatieganu" University of Medicine and Pharmacy, Department of Ophthalmology, Cluj-Napoca, Romania
[2]"Iuliu Hatieganu" University of Medicine and Pharmacy, Department of Medical Informatics and Biostatistics, Cluj-Napoca, Romania

Abstract

Purpose: The purpose of this study is to evaluate the outcomes of transpupillary diode laser photocoagulation for retinopathy of prematurity (ROP) in our hospital.

Methods: This is a retrospective case series that was carried out at the "Iuliu Hatieganu" University of Medicine and Pharmacy from Cluj-Napoca, Romania. The records of all the infants who received indirect diode laser photocoagulation for ROP, between January 1st 2006 – October 31st 2014 were reviewed. The following parameters were

* Corresponding author: simonanicoara1@gmail.com.

analized: gestational age, birth weight, postmenstrual age at treatment, postnatal age at treatment, type of pregnancy (unique or multiple), gender, number of laser sessions, ROP classification (zone and stage of the disease), postlaser evolution (regression or progression of ROP). The statistical analysis was performed with the program SPSS 22.0.

Results: During the above mentioned period of time, we performed diode laser photocoagulation for ROP in 168 eyes of 87 infants: 48 males (55.20%) and 39 females (44.80%). Gestational age was between 24 and 33 weeks (mean 28.67 weeks ± 2 weeks SD) and birth weight was between 600 and 1700 grams (mean 1123.33 grams ± 276.41grams SD). The postnatal age at treatment was between 5 and 13 weeks (mean 8.41weeks ± 1.97 weeks SD) and the postmenstrual age at treatment was between 32 and 41weeks (mean 37.10 weeks ± 1.77 weeks SD). We classified the 168 treated eyes into two categories: classic disease (stage 3+ ROP in zones 1 or 2) – 138 eyes (82.14%) and aggressive posterior ROP (AP-ROP) – 30 eyes (17.85%). ROP regressed in 148 eyes (88.09%). The success rate was significantly better in the classic ROP (95.65%) as compared to AP-ROP (53.33%).

Discussion: The rationale for the use of laser in ROP is discussed. The factors that influenced the ROP regression are analyzed, as follows: individual factors (ROP category, birth weight, gestational age, type of pregnancy, sex of the infant), timing of the laser treatment (postmenstrual age, postnatal age).

Conclusion: Indirect diode laser photocoagulation proved its efficacy in the treatment of ROP: in 88.58% of the treated eyes ROP regressed and the retina remained attached.

Introduction

Retinopathy of Prematurity (ROP) is a potentially blinding disease of the preterm infants [1]. Timely recognition and treatment of ROP are crucial for preventing blindness related to it. ROP is referred to as 2 types: type 1 ROP requires treatment and type 2 ROP must be followed up [2]. Laser photocoagulation of the retina aims to destroy the nonvascularized retina, in order to suppress the source of neovascularization. The goal of retinal laser ablation is to minimize unnecessary retinal destruction in cases that would regress spontaneously and to maximize the number of cases in which treatment prevents progression to retinal detachment [2]. The Ophthalmology and Neonatology Departments belonging to the "Iuliu Hatieganu" University of Medicine and Pharmacy from Cluj-Napoca, Romania, joined the ROP National Screening Program in 2005 and the laser treatment became available from 2006 on. In this chapter we aim to present the outcome of transpupillary diode laser photocoagulation for ROP performed in our hospital.

Material. Methods

This is a retrospective case series.

Setting

We performed this study at the "Iuliu Hatieganu" University of Medicine and Pharmacy from Cluj-Napoca, Romania. We carried out all the laser therapies in the Neonatology Department. The informed consent from the parents/tutors was obtained before the enrollment of the patients and the study has the approval of the Ethics Committee belonging to the "Iuliu Hatieganu" University of Medicine and Pharmacy.

Study Sample

We reviewed the records of all the infants who received indirect diode laser photocoagulation for ROP, between January 1st 2006 – October 31st 2014. In Romania, the screening for ROP is performed according to the following criteria: GA less/equal to 33 weeks and BW less/equal to 1500 grams. We also included in the screening for ROP, the premature infants with GA more than 33 weeks and BW more than 1500 grams, if other risk factors were associated: prolonged oxygen administration with saturation over 93%, repetead transfusions, sepsis, more than 6 days of mechanical ventilation for the cardio-respiratory support.

ROP Classification

We included each ROP case in a certain category on the ground of the ICROP revisited classification scheme [3]. This keeps the ICROP elaborated in 1984, taking into account the zone, the extension, the stage and the presence/absence of “plus” disease [4] and it adds to it the definition of "pre-plus" disease and of the aggressive posterior ROP (AP-ROP) [3]. AP-ROP is characterized by: posterior location, very severe plus disease, marked dilation and tortuosity of vessels in the posterior pole in all four quadrants with shunts between vessels within the retina. There is no well defined ridge, hemorrhages may be present at the junction between the vascularized and non-vascularized retina. AP-ROP may also appear as a flat neovascular network at the junction between the vascular and avascular retina [1].

Medical Intervention

We indicated the laser treatment in our series in the following circumstances: zone II stage 3 ROP, zone I stage 3 ROP and AP-ROP. In stage 3 zones I and II ROP, the laser was performed within 48 hours from the diagnosis and in AP-ROP, within 24 hours from the diagnosis. All the laser treatments were undertaken in the Neonatology Unit, under sedation. Prior the laser, we dilated the pupils with tropicamide 0.5% and phenylephrine 2.5%. We used a transpupillary portable diode laser, with the emission of 810 nm. We kept the eyes of the infants open during laser delivery with a lid speculum and we visualized the retina with a +28 diopters lens. In order to get access to the peripheral retina, we used a scleral depressor. We applied 200 ms, 150 - 400 mW laser spots in a near confluent manner, on all the surface of the avascular retina. This was achieved by placing the laser burns 0.25 burn width apart. We performed the first review 6 - 7 days after the treatment and we repeated the examination every 5 - 6 days, until there was evidence of ROP regression. If at the first review ROP showed signs of progression, laser treatment was completed the next day. We performed retreatment in the following circumstances: in eyes with persistent plus disease, active stage 3 disease, high ridge, localized tractional retinal detachment. We monitored all the eyes at a frequency dictated by the clinical condition to determine the risk of sequels.

Statistical Analysis

We performed statistical analysis with Microsoft Excel and SPSS software (version 22.0). Data are presented as mean ± standard deviation (SD) for the quantitative variables and as absolute and relative frequencies for categorical variables. Shapiro-Wilk test for normality, Levene's test for equality of variances, ANOVA test or the non-parametric Mann -Whitney U test for equality of means were used. Differences between the expected and the observed frequencies were assessed with the chi-square test. If the conditions for this test were not reached, the Fisher's exact test was used. P values less than 0.05 were regarded as significant.

Results

Clinical Characteristics of the Study Sample

During January 1st 2006 – October 31st 2014 we performed laser for ROP in 168 eyes belonging to 87 premature infants. Of the 87 premature infants, 48 (55.20%) were males and 39 (44.80%) were females. Of the 87 treated infants, 27 (31.03%) were from Cluj and 60 (68.96%) were referred to us from neighbouring departments where the laser treatment was not available. Of the 87 premature infants, 57 (65.50%) came from single pregnancies and 30 (34.50%), from multiple ones. The GA was between 24 and 33 weeks (mean 28.67 weeks ± 2 weeks SD) and the BW was between 600 and 1700 grams (mean 1123.33 grams ± 276.41 grams SD). The PNA at treatment was between 5 and 13 weeks (mean 8.41 weeks ± 1.97 weeks SD) and the PMA at treatment was between 32 and 41weeks (mean 37.10 weeks ± 1.77 weeks SD). All the above mentioned data are summarized in Table 1.

Table 1. Data of the lasered premature infants

Gender	
Males	48 (55.20%)
Females	39 (44.80%)
City of origin	
Cluj	27 (31.03%)
Outside Cluj	60 (68.96%)
Type of pregnancy	
Single	57 (65.50%)
Multiple	30 (34.50%)
GA (weeks)	28.67 ± 2
BW (grams)	1123.33 ± 276.41
Mean PNA at treatment (weeks)	8.41 ± 1.97
Mean PMA at treatment (weeks)	37.10 ± 1.77

Classification of ROP in Our Series

Classification of ROP in our series is presented in Table 2.

Table 2. ROP classification in our series

ROP classification	Eyes (number)	Eyes (%)
Stage II zone 2	3	1.73
Stage III zone 2	118	68.20
Stage III zone 1	20	11.56
AP-ROP	30	17.34
Stage IV A	1	0.57
Stage V	1	0.57

We performed laser photocoagulation for ROP in 168 eyes, belonging to the following categories: stage III zone 2 ROP, stage III zone 1 ROP and AP-ROP. Retinal laser photocoagulation was bilateral in 81 cases and unilateral in 6 cases. The reasons for unilateral laser treatment were: stage II zone 2 ROP (3 eyes), stage IV A ROP (1 eye), stage V ROP (1 eye) and congenital atrophy (1 eye). We followed the eyes with stage II zone 2 ROP every 3 days and they all regressed spontaneously, with no need of laser treatment.

Timing of the Laser Treatment for ROP

We defined the moment of treatment by two parameters: PNA and PMA at treatment.

The PNA at treatment varied between 5 - 13 weeks in our series (mean 8.41 weeks ± 1.97 weeks SD). The mean PNA in the favorable outcome group was 8.47 weeks and in the unfavorable outcome group the mean PNA was 7.40 weeks. The difference is statistically significant ($p = 0.031$, non-parametric Mann-Whitney U test). The treatment was performed at PNA less/equal to 8 weeks in 94 eyes (55.95%) and at more than 8 weeks after birth in 74 eyes (44.04%). Within the group treated at PNA less/equal to 8 weeks, ROP regressed in 80 eyes (85.10%). If the treatment was performed at more than 8 weeks after birth, ROP regressed in 68 eyes (91.89%). This difference is not statistically significant (chi-square test $p = 0.188$).

The PMA at treatment varied between 32 – 41 weeks (mean 37.10 weeks ± 1.77 weeks SD). The mean PMA at treatment in the favorable outcome group was 36.55 weeks and in the unfavorable outcome group, 37.12 weeks. The difference is not statistically significant (ANOVA test $p = 0.172$). PMA at treatment was less/equal to 37 weeks in 94 eyes (55.95%) and more than 37 weeks in 74 eyes (44.04%). Within the group with PMA at treatment less/equal to 37 weeks, ROP regressed after the laser treatment in 83 eyes (88.29%) and in the cases with PMA at treatment of more than 37 weeks (74 eyes), the laser treatment induced ROP regression in 65 eyes (87.83%). The difference is not statistically significant (chi-square test $p = 0.435$).

ROP Regression after the Laser Therapy

We registered ROP regression after the laser photocoagulation in 148 of the 168 treated eyes (88.09%). Laser was performed in one session in 133 eyes (89.86%) and in two sessions in 15 eyes (10.13%), of which 10 were with AP-ROP (66.66%). Macular dragging was identified in 5 of the 148 (3.37%) eyes with the retina attached after the laser therapy. They all belonged to the AP-ROP type.

The complications related to the laser therapy were represented by six cases of mild anterior uveitis, 5 in AP-ROP and one in zone I stage 3 ROP. They responded promptly to mydriatic and antiinflammatory eye drops.

Individual Factors Associated with the Outcomes of Laser Therapy

We analyzed the following individual factors in relationship with the outcomes of the laser therapy: ROP type, gender, type of pregnancy, BW and GA.

Within the stage 3 zone II ROP group (118 eyes), the laser photocoagulation of the nonvascularized retina was followed by ROP involution in 113 eyes (95.76%) and ROP progression in 5 eyes (4.23%). Among the 20 eyes with stage 3 zone I ROP, the postlaser regression of ROP was noted in 19 eyes (95%) and the worsening of ROP in 1 eye (5%). In the group of 30 eyes with AP-ROP, the laser induced the ROP regression in 16 eyes (53.33%) and the ROP progression in 14 eyes (46.66%). The statistical tests proved that the outcome of the laser treatment was significantly worse in AP-ROP as compared to stage 3 zone II ROP and stage 3 zone I ROP.

Statistically, the difference is very significant (corrected chi square p = 0.000 and Fisher exact test p = 0.000). These data are summarized in Table 3.

Table 3. Regression after the laser treatment according to the ROP classification

ROP classification	Eyes with regression (number)	Eyes with regression (%)
Stage 3 zone II	113	95.76
Stage 3 zone I	19	95.00
AP-ROP	16	53.33

ROP failed to regress after the laser treatment in 11 of the 90 eyes belonging to the male gender (12.22%) and in 9 of the 78 eyes belonging to the female gender (11.53%). The difference is not statistically significant (chi square test p = 0.870, Fisher exact test p = 1.000). Of the108 eyes belonging to infants coming from single pregnancies, the laser treatment was followed by ROP regression in 96 eyes (88.88%) and of the 60 eyes within the multiple pregnancies group, ROP regressed after the laser treatment in 52 eyes (86.66%). Statistically, the type of pregnancy did not influence significantly the result of the laser treatment (chi square test p = 0.641, Fisher exact test p = 0.627).

The mean BW in the group with favorable outcome after laser therapy was 1102.16 grams, whereas in the group with unfavorable outcome it was 1232.00 grams. This difference is statistically significant (p = 0.046, ANOVA test). Within the 168 treated eyes, 64 belonged to premature infants having the BW of less/equal to 1000 grams (38.09%) and 104, to premature infants having the BW of more than 1000 grams (61.90%). ROP failed to regress after the laser therapy in 4 eyes (6.25%) from the first group and in 16 eyes (15.38%) from the second group. There is a tendency towards statistical significance (Chi square test p = 0.059 and Fisher test p = 0.086).

The mean GA in the group with unfavorable outcome (20 eyes) was 29.25 weeks, whereas in the group with favorable outcome it was 28.58 weeks. The difference is not statistically significant (p = 0.162, ANOVA test). Among the 168 treated eyes, the GA was less/equal to 28 weeks in 90 eyes (53.57%) and more than 28 weeks in 78 eyes (46.42%). Within the group of GA less/equal to 28 weeks, ROP regressed after the laser treatment in 83 eyes (92.22%) and within the group of premature infants born after more than 28 weeks of gestation, ROP regressed following laser photocoagulation in 65 eyes

(83.33%). The evaluation of cases distribution according to GA ($\leq$ 28 weeks or > 28 weeks) proves a tendency towards statistical significance (Fisher test: $p = 0.095$).

Discussion

Rationale of the Laser Treatment for ROP

ROP is a two phase disease, possibly preceded by an antenatal phase of retinal sensitisation via inflammation. Phase 1 is characterized by oxygen toxicity and phase 2, by hypoxia-mediated vasoproliferation [2]. In phase 1, when the immature retina of the preterm babies is exposed to high levels of oxygen, the pro-angiogenic growth factors (such as Vascular Endothelial Growth Factor - VEGF) decrease with subsequent cessation of vessel growth. In phase 2, the relative hypoxia that was generated in phase 1 leads to higher VEGF levels and the forming of new vessels [5, 6]. Laser photocoagulation destroys the VEGF producing cells and VEGF-inducing cytokines. The decrease in plasma levels of all these angiogenic factors following laser photocoagulation may be attributed to laser treatment [7].

The role of laser in ROP is to destroy the non-vascularized retina in order to remove the source of angiogenic factors [8, 9]. Laser photocoagulation destroys the cells that produce VEGF and also the VEGF-inducing cytokines. The decrease in plasma levels of all these angiogenic factors following laser photocoagulation may be attributed to laser treatment [7].

Laser versus Cryotherapy in the Treatment of ROP

Ablation of the avascular retina proved its efficacy in preventing blindness by ROP for the first time in 1988 with cryo [10]. Later, in 1994, the laser ROP study group showed that the destruction of the avascular retina with laser is better than cryo, as it was associated with less severe side effects [11]. Transpupillary laser photocoagulation of the retina has replaced cryotherapy for ROP, because of better visual outcomes and fewer side effects [2].

It has advantages over cryotherapy: it is more convenient and technically easier, the treatment is more precise and less traumatic, it avoids lesions to the external eye [1].

A study showed better structural and functional outcome at 10 years of laser compared to cryotherapy [12]. According to the results of this study, cryotherapy was associated with 7.2 more macular dragging than laser [12]. The mean best corrected visual acuity was 20/66 in the laser group, as compared with 20/182 in eyes treated with cryotherapy [12]. The laser treated eyes were significantly less myopic as the eyes treated with cryotherapy, as proven by the mean spherical equivalent of -4.48 D in the laser treated eyes, as compared to -7.65 D in the eyes that had undergone cryotherapy [12].

Disadvantages of Laser for the Treatment of ROP

Near confluent laser treatment is the standard of care for ROP but it has the disadvantage of being destructive. Also the retinal vessels never continue their growth beyond the treatment zone. One of the long term complications associated with laser treatment, especially in zone I ROP, is the significant loss of visual field. The studies that showed no effect or little effect of laser on the visual field were performed on zone II ROP cases. Myopia can occur, especially following repeated laser treatments for zone I ROP. Axial myopia develops due to scleral weakening. Sometimes, after extensive laser for zone I ROP, cystoid macular edema was noted [13].

Timing of the Laser Treatment for ROP

ROP can be regarded as a model of acute retinal neovascularization. By consequence, the window of opportunity during which treatment is effective is very short. Timing is crucial for obtaining good outcomes following laser photocoagulation and it is strictly related to the screening for ROP. For the screening to be correct, knowing the natural evolution of ROP in correlation with time is essential. Usually, ROP does not develop during the first 2 weeks after birth. PMA is more accurate than PNA for the description of ROP evolution [2]. Stage 1 ROP is detected around 34 weeks PMA, pre-threshold ROP - around 36 weeks PMA and threshold ROP - around 37 weeks PMA. The retina has a complete vascularization by 40 – 44 weeks PMA. Therefore, the interval for ROP detection is between 32 – 40 weeks PMA. The critical phase, during which ROP progresses and may have to be treated, is between 34 – 37 weeks PMA [14, 15].

The mean PMA at treatment in our series was 37.10 weeks, at the superior limit of the above mentioned interval. Even if in our series the mean PMA at treatment in the favorable outcome group was lower than in the unfavorable outcome group (36.55 weeks versus 37.12 weeks), this difference was not statistically significant. Also, the infants who were treated at PMA ≤ 37 weeks were not more likely to have a better outcome as those treated at PMA > 37 weeks.

Paradoxically, in the favorable outcome group the mean PNA at treatment was significantly higher than in the unfavorable outcome group (8.47 weeks versus 7.40 weeks). This proves that PNA at treatment is not the best timing indicator for assessing the outcome. Also, the infants treated within 8 weeks from birth in our series were not more likely to have a better outcome as those treated more than 8 weeks after birth, according to the statistic analysis.

Technique and Complications of the Laser Therapy for ROP

The regression rate of ROP following laser on our series was 88.09%, which is comparable to the ones we found in the litterature [1, 11, 15, 16]. We applied the laser spots on all the surface of the avascular retina, from the anterior margin of the ridge to the ora serrata, in a near confluent manner, as the scars will expand [17]. In order to avoid the anterior segment ischemia that may be caused by ablating the long cilliary arteries, we used a less confluent pattern of laser photocoagulation in the clock hours corresponding to the horizontal meridian [18]. It was proved that a dense pattern of laser photocoagulation was more successful than a less dense pattern in reducing the disease progression [19]. There is not a direct correlation between the covered area and the number of laser burns, as the size of the laser burn varies according to the distance of the lens from the eye, the dioptric power of the lens, the laser burn intensity and duration. Therefore, the most useful guide to the amount of treatment is the adequate coverage, not the number of laser burns [17].

In 4 eyes we placed laser burns also posterior to the ridge, as recommended by several authors [18]. We had two reasons for using this technique: to create focal chorio-retinal adhesions in order to limit the spread of tractional retinal detachment and to destroy the ischemic areas known to occur in this location. All the 4 eyes had a good anatomical outcome. Other authors do not recommend the application of laser burns posterior to the ridge, arguing that it potentially reduces the peripheral visual field with no proven benefit [15].

Macular dragging was identified in 5 cases of AP-ROP. This condition prevents the normal development of the visual acuity by displacing the macula.

In all our cases we delivered the laser energy transpupillary. Laser energy can be delivered also through the sclera. The two delivery methods have the same efficacy, but the transscleral approach is more traumatic, although it has the advantage of decreasing the risk of cataract formation (by circumventing the lens) [15]. In our series we had no case of cataract formation with the transpupillary laser delivery system. If argon green light is used, since it is absorbed by blood vessels, the risk of burns to the tunica vasculosa lentis and the adjacent lens is higher than with the infrared diode laser [1, 15, 20]. Beside cataract, other complications were reported with laser: cornea and iris burns, hyphema, retinal hemorrhages, choroidal ruptures [1]. The only complication related to the laser treatment in our series was the mild anterior uveitis noted in 6 cases, 5 AP-ROP and 1 zone I stage 3+, probably provoqued by the high degree of energy that was delivered into the eyes [21].

Influence of the Individual Factors on the Outcomes after Laser Therapy

We are going to discuss the following factors in relation with the outcome of laser treatment in ROP: classic ROP or AP-ROP, sex of the infant, type of pregnancy (unique or multiple), BW and GA.

We included in the category of "classic" ROP the eyes with zones I and II, stage 3+ disease. In classic ROP, regression rate was around 95%, whereas in AP-ROP, the disease regressed in only 53.33% of cases following laser treatment (Table 3). The statistical tests proved that AP-ROP was significantly less likely to regress after laser as compared to classic ROP in our series. Several studies reported poor outcome after laser treatment in AP-ROP [22-26]. Early and aggressive confluent laser photocoagulation optimized the outcomes, but some eyes still progress to retinal detachment [1]. Moreover, of the 15 eyes that needed two laser sessions, 10 were with AP-ROP (66.66%). AP-ROP progresses rapidly, circumferentially, usually not through the classic stages 1 to 3 and therefore it may be missed by an unexperienced examiner [1]. Any delay in the diagnosis and treatment of this severe form of ROP has disastrous consequences. In the AP-ROP cases, the difficulty comes also from the fact that the laser treatment has to be performed immediately, before any ridge develops. The absence of any landmark makes the laser photocoagulation very difficult [3, 4]. The lack of macular development at this age adds more challenge to these cases [25, 27, 28].

There are publications reporting higher rate of visual impairment by ROP in males as compared to females which is presumed to be related to the relative maturation of the lungs and central nervous system in boys [29]. In our study, the male gender was not associated with a poorer outcome after the laser treatment for ROP.

The type of pregnancy (unique or multiple) had no significant influence on the outcome of laser for ROP in our series.

BW was reported to be a bad prognosis factor for ROP evolution after laser [30]. Our study proves the contrary: the mean BW in the unfavorable outcome group was significantly higher than in the favorable outcome group. When we analyze the outcome according to BW ≤ or > than 1000 grams, the results are not statistically significant.

Our results show that GA was not significanlty associated with the outcome of laser treatment for ROP in our series.

The results of our research prove that the only factor that influenced very significantly the results of the laser treatment was the ROP category. The outcomes were very significantly worse in AP-ROP as compared to the classic ROP. The overall ROP regression rate after transpupillary diode laser photocoagulation was good on our series: 88.09%. However, the disappointing results of the laser ablation of the non-vascularized retina in AP-ROP (53.33% regression rate) motivated us to replace it by intravitreal injections with anti-VEGF agents. As such, during the last 6 years, our therapy of choice in AP-ROP is represented by intravitreal injections with anti-VEGF.

Conclusion

Indirect diode laser photocoagulation of the retina proved its efficacy and safety in the treatment of ROP in our series. ROP regressed following laser treatment in 88.09% of the cases. We report only a few mild anterior uveities following laser treatment that responded promptly to treatment with no sequels. AP-ROP was significantly less likely to regress after laser therapy as compared to the classic form of ROP (zones I and II, stage 3+). Mean BW in the group with favorable outcome was significantly lower than in the group with unfavorable outcome. Mean PNA at treatment was significantly lower in the unfavorable outcome group, as compared to the favorable outcome group. GA, sex, type of pregnancy, PMA at treatment did not influence significantly the outcome of laser photocoagulation for ROP in our series.

References

[1] Clark, D. & Mandal, K. (2008). Treatment of retinopathy of prematurity. *Early Human Development, 84,* 95 – 99.

[2] Hellström, Ann & Smith, Lois E.H. & Dammann, O.(2013). Retinopathy of prematurity. *Lancet, 382,* 1445 – 1457.

[3] Drenser, K.A.& Trese, M.T.& Capone, A. Jr. (2010). Aggressive posterior retinopathy of prematurity. *Retina, 30,*S37-S40.

[4] Axer-Siegel, R.& Snir, M.& Cotlear, D. et al. (2008). Diode laser treatment of posterior retinopathy of prematurity. *Br J Ophthalmol*, *84*, 1383-1386.

[5] Mintz-Hittner, H.A.& Kennedy, K.A.& Chuang, A. (2011). Efficacy of intravitreal Bevacizumab for stage 3+ retinopathy of prematurity. *N Engl J Med, 364,* 603-615.

[6] Soh, Y.& Fujino, T.& Hatsukawa, Y.(2008). Progression and Timing of Treatment of Zone I Retinopathy of Prematurity. *Am J Ophthalmol, 146,* 369 –374.

[7] Imamoglu, E.Y.& Gunay, M.& Gursoy T. et al. (2014). Effect of laser photocoagulation on plasma levels of VEGF-A, VEGFR-2, and Tie2 in infants with retinopathy of prematurity. *J AAPOS, 18,* 466-470.

[8] O'Keefe, M.& Kirwan, C. (2008). Screening for retinopathy of prematurity, *Early Human Development*, *84*, 89–94.

[9] O'Keefe, M.& Kirwan, C. (2006). Diode laser versus cryotherapy in treatment of ROP. *BJO, 90,* 402–403.

[10] Cryotherapy for Retinopathy of Prematurity Cooperative Group (1998). Multicenter trial of cryotherapy for retinopathy of prematurity. Preliminary results. *Arch Ophthalmol, 106,* 471–479.

[11] Essex, R. W.& Carden, S. M. & Elder, J. E. (2005) Two-year results of laser treatment for retinopathy of prematurity at a single neonatal intensive care unit, *Clinical & Experimental Ophthalmology*, *33*, 390–394.

[12] Ng, E.Y.J.& Connolly, B.P. & McNamara, A. & Regillo, C.&Vander, J.F. & Tasmad, W. (2002). A comparison of laser photocoagulation with cryotherapy for threshold retinopathy of prematurity at 10 years. Part 1. Visual function and structural outcome. *Ophthalmology, 109*, 928–935.

[13] Mintz-Hittner, H.A.(2012). Treatment of retinopathy of prematurity with vascular endothelial growth factor inhibitors. *Early Human Development, 88,* 937-941.

[14] Good, W.V. & Carden, S.M. (2006). Retinopathy of prematurity, *Br J Ophthalmol*, *90*, 254-255.

[15] Kieselbach, G. F.& Ramharter, A.& Baldissera, I. & Kralinger, M. T. (2006). Laser photocoagulation for retinopathy of prematurity: structural and functional outcome. *Acta Ophthalmologica Scandinavica, 84*, 21–26.

[16] Fallaha, N.& Lynn, M.J.& Aaberg, T.M. Jr. & Lambert, S.R. (2002). Clinical outcome of confluent laser photoablation for retinopathy of prematurity, *J AAPOS, 6,*81-85.

[17] Rezai, K.A. & Elliott, D. & Ferrone, P.J. & Kim, R.W. (2005). Near confluent laser photocoagulation for the treatment of threshold retinopathy of prematurity. *Arch Ophthalmol*, *123,* 621–626.

[18] Kaiser, R.S.& Trese, M.T.(2001). Iris atrophy, cataracts, and hypotony following peripheral ablation for threshold retinopathy of prematurity. *Arch of Ophthalmol, 119*, 615–617.

[19] Banach, M.J.& Ferrone, P.J.& Trese, M.T. (2000). A comparison of dense versus less dense diode laser photocoagulation patterns for threshold retinopathy of prematurity. *Ophthalmology, 107,* 324–328.

[20] Salgado, C.M. & Celik, Y.& Vanderveen, D.K. (2010). Anterior Segment Complications After Diode Laser Photocoagulation for Prethreshold Retinopathy of Prematurity, *Am J Ophthalmol,150*, 6 – 9.

[21] Nicoara, S.D. & Cristian, C. & Irimescu, I. & Stefanut, A.C. & Zaharie, G. (2014). Diode Laser Photocoagulation for Retinopathy of Prematurity: Outcomes After 7 Years of Treatment. *J Pediatr Ophthalmol Strabismus, 51,* 39 – 45.

[22] Sanghi, G. & Dogra, M.R.& Das, P.& Vinekar, A.& Gupta, A & Dutta, S. (2009). Aggressive posterior retinopathy of prematurity in Asian Indian babies: spectrum of disease and outcome after laser treatment. *Retina*, *29,* 1335–1339.

[23] Drenser, K.A.& Trese, M.T.& Capone, A. Jr. (2010). Aggressive posterior retinopathy of prematurity. *Retina 30 (4 Suppl)*, S37–40.

[24] Jalali, S.& Kesarwani, S& Hussain, A.(2011). Outcomes of a protocol based management for zone 1 retinopathy of prematurity: the Indian Twin Cities ROP Screening Program report number 2. *Am J Ophthalmol, 151,*719–724.
[25] Kychenthal, A.& Dorta, P& Katz, X. (2006). Zone I retinopathy of prematurity: clinical characteristics and treatment outcomes. *Retina, 26(7 Suppl)*, S11–15.
[26] Azuma, N.& Ishikawa, K.& Hama, Y & Hiraoka, M & Suzuki, Y & Nishina, S. (2006). Early vitreous surgery for aggressive posterior retinopathy of prematurity. *AmJ Ophthalmol, 142*, 636–643.
[27] O'Keefe, M. & Lanigan, B. & Long V.W. (2003). Outcomes of zone I retinopathy of prematurity. *Acta Ophthalmol Scand, 81*, 614-616.
[28] Récsán, Z. & Vámos, R. & Salacz, G. (2003). Laser treatment of zone I prethreshold and stage 3 threshold retinopathy of prematurity. *J Pediatr Ophthalmol Strabismus, 40*, 204-207.
[29] Cole, C.H.(2010). Making Sense of Clinical Determinants of Retinopathy of Prematurity. *The Journal of Pediatrics, 157*, 4-7.
[30] Coats, D.K. & Miller, A.M. & Hussein, M.A.W. & Brady, Mc Creery, K.M. & Holz E.& Paysse, E.A. (2005). Involution of retinopathy of prematurity after laser treatment: factors associated with development of retinal detachment. *Am J Ophthalmol, 140,* 214–222.

In: Retinopathy of Prematurity (ROP)
Editor: Elmira Aguilar
ISBN: 978-1-63482-644-0

Chapter 6

Late Complications of Retinopathy of Prematurity

Monika Ecsedy [*] ***and Zsuzsa Recsan***
Budapest Department of Ophthalmology,
Semmelweis University, Hungary

Abstract

Retinopathy of prematurity is a lifelong disease. Compared to full term population, higher prevalence of refractive errors, amblyopia, stabismus, reduction in visual field, impaired color vision and contrast sensitivity is found. Preterm delivery resulted in a disrupted development of both anterior and posterior segment of the eye. Preterm birth showed a significant impact on axial length, keratometry values, corneal thickness, lower and higher order refractive errors of the cornea. The anterior segment parameters such as shallower anterior chamber depth and thicker lens were determined by the presence of retinopathy in the acute phase. In the posterior segment, higher foveal thickness was found compared to full-term subjects. The impairment of normal centrifugal movement of foveal cone nuclei and inner retinal cells is supposed. Pigment disturbances, macular dragging due to regressed retinopathy in the periphery, developmental restriction of optic nerve head, thinner choroid are associated with worse best corrected visual acuity in formerly preterm

[*] E-mail: ecsedy@yahoo.co.uk.

patient. Due to the peripheral degenerative changes in the retina, abnormal vitreoretinal interface, retinal detachment either rhegmatogeneous or tractional can develop not only in acute phase of ROP but in the late adulthood, as well.

Introduction

Preterm birth itself and retinopathy of prematurity (ROP) have both been reported to impact the developing visual system, resulting in not temporary but permanent deficits which persist into later childhood [1] and even adult life [2] It is already well known that infants born at less than 32 weeks' gestation are not only at high risk of retinopathy of prematurity in the first months of their life,but they can also suffer from long-term refractive errors, amblyopia, strabismus, and optic nerve abnormalities, linked to the degree of prematurity and the presence of cerebral damage [3-5]. Ocular growth or emmetropisation procedure is different in this preterm population from those in children born at full term [6, 7]. It is also not uncommon for adolescents with a history of mild retinopathy of prematurity (ROP) to have mild deficits in letter acuity that cannot be corrected by careful refraction, even in the absence of clinical ROP in the macula and the absence of early high refractive errors [8]. But until recent times we did not know a lot about the background of all these phenomena. In the last two decades new non-invasive diagnostic methodes-such as optical coherence tomography (OCT) or Sheimpflug imaging (Pentacam)-helped us to examine, and better understand the subtle structural anomalies and functional deficits that may persist years after clinical ROP resolves.

Ocular Growth and Refractive Error Development in Premature Infants

Ocular structures go through a continuous development and remodeling process before and after birth. Premature departure from the intrauterine environment may affect ocular development or later emmetropization, so refractive status of the eye [9]. Myopia is certainly the most studied in the literature [6-12]. It has been linked to preterm birth (birth weight and gestational age may be independent risk factors) and separately to retinopathy of prematurity and its treatment [10-12]. Both the prevalence and the magnitude of myopia enlarge with increasing severity of ROP and are greater in treated eyes compared to eyes not required treatment. In addition prematurely born children also tend to develop other refractive errors, such as hyperopia, astigmatism and anisometropia [9].

The most common method for measuring details of the anterior segment and axial bulbus length used in the literature was ultrasound (US) biometry; however, this technique requires a contact device and precise measurement depends on correct probe alignment and centration [10-12]. Rotating Scheimpflug photography (Pentacam) is a relatively new technique, that images the entire anterior segment from the anterior corneal surface to the posterior lens surface, with good reproducibility and repeatability [13-16]. It assesses the curvature and elevation of the anterior and posterior corneal surfaces, pachymetry maps, the anterior chamber depth (ACD) and the anterior chamber angle [17-23]. Pentacam is also able to measure lower and higher order aberrations of the entire cornea and its front and back surface. These data are presented as lower order and higher order root mean square errors (RMS LOA and RMS HOA), including the third up to the eighth Zernike orders.

Ultrasound reports suggested that myopia was mainly influenced by anterior segment components such as anterior chamber depth and lens thickness. Majima and Hibino reported that children with retinal residua of ROP had myopia as a result of a combination of increased lens thickness, and decreased anterior chamber depth [24]. Donzis et al. found that myopia was caused by high crystalline lens power and Hittner et al. demonstrated shallowing of the anterior chamber in myopic eyes when residua of ROP was found on fundus examination [25, 26]. Whereas hyperopia was mainly attributable to shorter axial length, while astigmatism was primarily cornea-related [9].

Our study group also found a shallower anterior segment and a significantly thicker lens with shorter axial bulbus length with Pentacam, in a cohort of preterm born children, 7-14 years of age, with good final central vision, who had moderate ROP or even no retinopathy during the neonatal period. We also demonstrated that anterior segment parmeters show graeter variability, and anterior chamber depth and lens thickness do not correlate in premature children while a moderate negative correlation can be observed in controls (Figure 1) [27]. The ratio between the anterior segment depth of the eye and the axial length was significantly higher in the preterm group compared to controls (Figure 2) [27]. Modified early emmetropisation process [28] caused by the biological stress of early extrauterin enviroment and the developing retinopathy, may result in a more anteriorly positioned crystalline lens [10]. These findings suggest that an anterior segment growth arrest -which was described previously only for myopic preterm eyes in the ultrasound studies [29, 30], -exist also in hyperopic preterm born children. Additionally, the significantly higher anterior segment length/axial length ratio found in our preterm patients imply that in preterm eyes a tendence to emmetropisation exists: ie. shorter axial length may be a compensation for the anterior segment growth arrest. Another explanation could be, that this growth arrest manifests not only in the anterior segment but the whole eyeball.

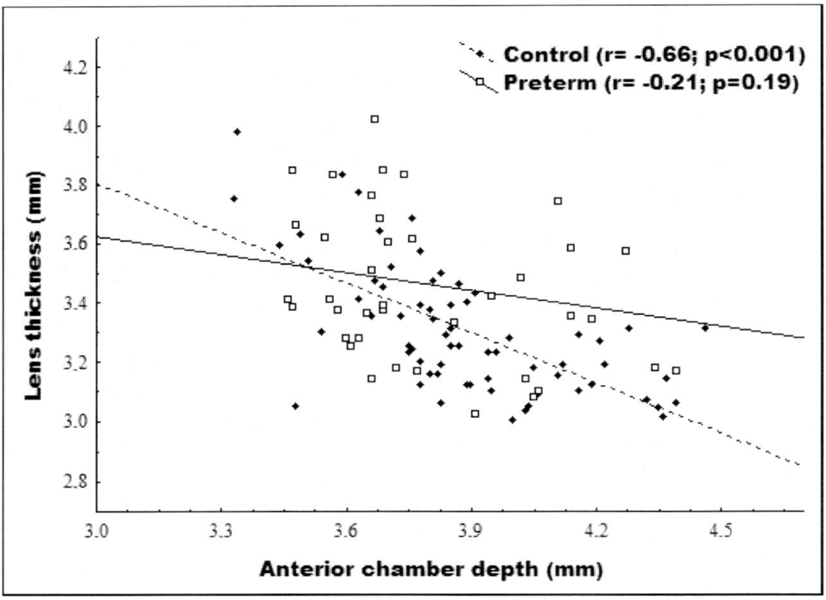

Figure 1. Linear regression demonstrating the correlation between lens thickness and anterior chamber depth (ACD) in the premature and in the control group.

Pentacam also showed an elevated corneal lower order aberrations and an even greater increase in corneal higher order aberrations -playing an important role in longterm refractive errors and visual disturbances-in preterm children compared to fullterm born classmates [27]. This suggests, that corneal morphology and developement may also be severely modified by premature birth or ROP. Fielder et al. nearly two decades ago postulated that the reduced temperature of the extrauterine eye leads to slowing of corneal growth, less flattening of the cornea [31]. The role of other factors such as light exposure and patterned visual stimulation on refractive development for short period before term are not well studied yet. Fledelius and Greisen found an increase in corneal curvature in low birthweight children regardless of ROP status [32]. Fledelius also described in a 7-9 year follow-up study, that the development of the anterior segment (corneal radius of curvature) was significantly influenced by the preterm delivery in patients with or without ROP [33]. At the same time Quinn observed a strong association between higher incidence of astigmatism and more severe ROP, however the gestational ages and birth weights of infants in the study were much lower than those of the infants in the present study [34].

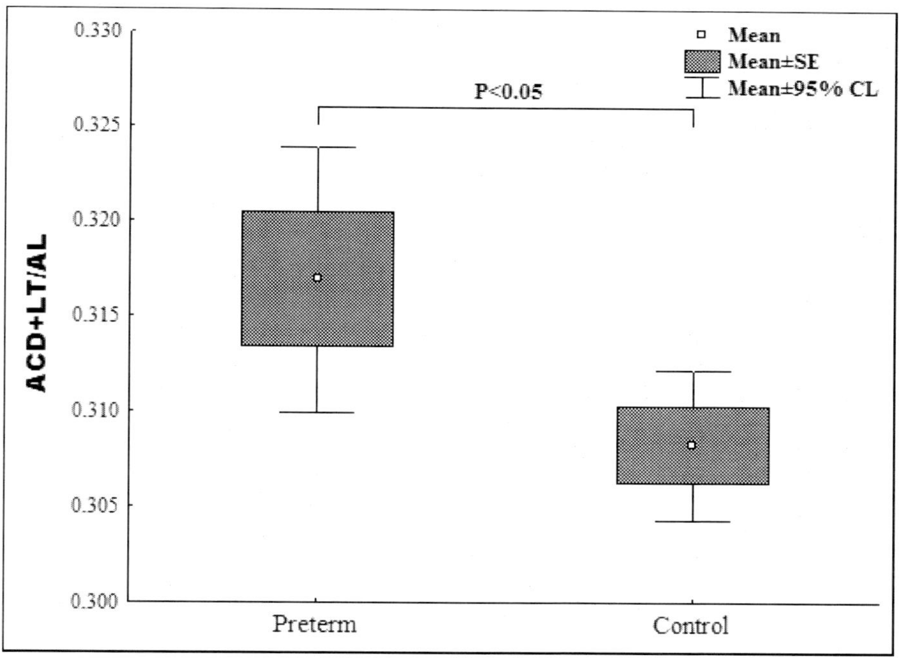

Figure 2. Ratio between the anterior segment of the eye (ACD+LT) and the axial length (AL) in the preterm group compared to controls.

By investigating the impact of the premature birth itself and the stage of retinopathy or laser treatment on anterior segment changes and axial length in our patients, we found that axial bulbus length and lens thickness depended on more of premature birth, while anterior chamber depth was rather depended on ROP stage. Laser treatment also showed a marginally significant impact on anterior chamber depth. Wether the forming retinopathy in the peripherial avascular retina may influence the lens position and cause anterior chamber shallowing is unknown.

Long-term Macular Morphological Changes in Formerly Preterm Children

Several animal studies [35, 36] investigating the development of the fovea suggested that ROP and prematurity itself alters the development of the central retina. Recent studies underlied this subtle macular dysfunction by using multifocal ERG for investigate ROP associated neural retinal development alterations [37] OCT imaging of the macular area is known to be highly reproducible and it is also found to be a useful tool for the measurement of macular volume, and foveal thickness [38, 39].

Optical coherence tomography investigation in 2007 by our study group demonstrated that ROP regressed with mild or no sequale was associated with a lower total macular volume, a thicker fovea and a thinner inner and outer macula compared to full term, healthy children. The foveal depression became smoth, cells' jam was observed. A thick layer was imaged between the lamina limitans interna and the photoreceptor layer and it corresponded to inner retinal layers. Foveal and central retinal thicknesses were significantly larger in eyes with ROP (ROP stage 1-3) than in control eyes. The values of these parameters in eyes of preterm children without ROP were between those of control group and of groupswith stage 1-3 ROP. The Mann-Whitney test showed a significant difference in the central retinal thickness of the three preterm groups compared with the control group. At the same time, the foveal thickness was similar in pretrm children without ROP and controls. The parafoveal region (inner and outer retinal thicknesses) in formerly preterm children did not differ significantly from full-term age matched volunteers. The thickened central region in formerly preterm children (groups with or without ROP) did not affect the value of the total macular volume, and it was not significantly higher than in the full-term group (Figure 3) [40].

One of the key findings of our study is that OCT imaging showed quantitative and qualitative modifications in the macular structure of formerly preterm children. The changes could reflect mainly the interrupted development of the eye. Small foveal avascular zone observed in a fluorescein angiographic and later in adaptive optics fourier domain OCT studies [41] performed on former preterm children could also support this idea.

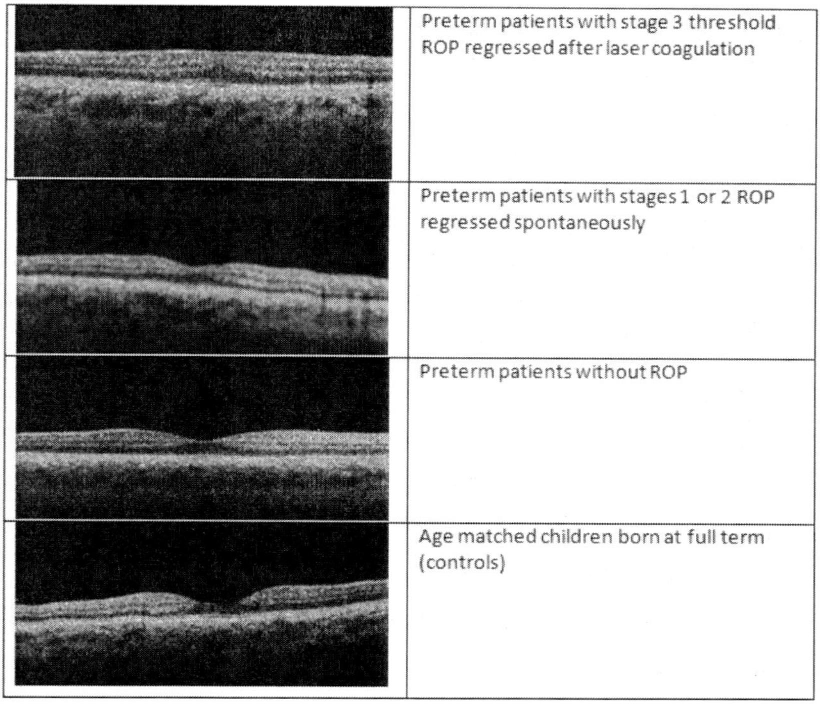

Figure 3. OCT scans of representative cases from premature patients with ROp stages 0-3. The central retinal thickness was the largest in group I, the mean values descended in group II and III toward to the values of group IV. The fovea is thickened, foveal depression is flattened in the groups I, II and III, the inner retinal layers seem to be continued above the photoreceptor layer. Group I: preterm patients with stage 3 threshold ROP regressed after laser coagulation, Group II: preterm patients with stages 1 or 2 ROP regressed spontaneously, Group III: preterm patients without ROP, Group IV: age matched children born at full term.

Foveal avascular zone was provided to be densely vascularized in developing humans. Normally, this fine meshwork undergoes regression by apoptosis. But it was detected that this process almost never occurs in children born before 30th gestational week [42]. Another possible proof could be served by electroretinographic studies. Significant deficits in amplitude and implicit time of mfERG responses have been recently published among children with a history of retinopathy of prematurity. Like bipolar cells make main contribution to the mfERG responses, the large discrepancy between the ROP and control amplitudes in the central rings raises the possibility that the difference in bipolar cell density is graetest in the central retina. Up to these findings the autors suspect that the developmental re-distribution of the central retina is altered in ROP subjects [11]. In normal foveal development, the diameter of the rod free zone decreases from approximatly 1400μm at 26 weeks gestation to 500μm in the mature eye as cone outer segments elongate and inner segments become more slender [35, 43, 44]. The foveal cone outer segments pack more tightly together, affording improved acuity [43, 44]. The foveal cone nuclei and inner retinal cells move away from the tightly packed foveal cone outer segments [45]. Thus as normal development proceeds, the distance from the center of the fovea to the cone photoreceptor nuclei and bipolar cells increases [45]. The decrease or absence of this migration in preterm babies can be an explanation, for the diminution of foveal depression and the continuity of bipolar and amacrin cell layer, seen on OCT scans.

Colour Vision, Contrast Sensitivity and Cone Function

Since the first description of tritan defects in preterm born infants by Abramov [46] a lot of study investigated color vision in this population with psychophysical methods [46-50] but they had controversal results. In the CRYO-ROP study, with pseudoisochromatic plates, they found an increased occurrence of blue-yellow deficits in children born before term, which was not related to birth weight, gestational age or severity of ROP, and showed no correlation with cryotherapy treatment [51]. The increased prevalence of impaired color vision, reported earlier in the CRYO-ROP study with the Standard Pseudoisochromatic Plates (SPP) in a big population [51], couldn't be detected after in several smaller studies with psychophisical methods [46-48, 50, 52]. We either couldn't detect any special color vision defect in 7-14 years old preterm born children with mild ROP; compared to controls with the Fansworth D15 and the Lantony desaturated (L15) tests [53]. We chose these two color vision tests because they are rather short, so easier for children, and L15 was found to be the most suitable test for screening of early color vision abnormalities in uncomplicated juvenile diabetes [54]. According to the literature, the SPP test used in the CRYO-ROP study, demonstrated low sensitivity in early color vision defects in diabetes patients [54].

Recent ERG studies showed that ROP has an effect on the photoreceptors and post receptor retina that persist even after its active phase. The late-maturing central retina and particularly the rod outer segments in the macula, appear to be vulnerable to these effects. Subtle deficits also occur in peripheral retinal function and persist into adolescence and early adulthood [55-58]. According to Fulton et al. ROP has less effect on the cone than on the rod photoresponses suggesting that cones are more resistant to the ROP disease process [59].

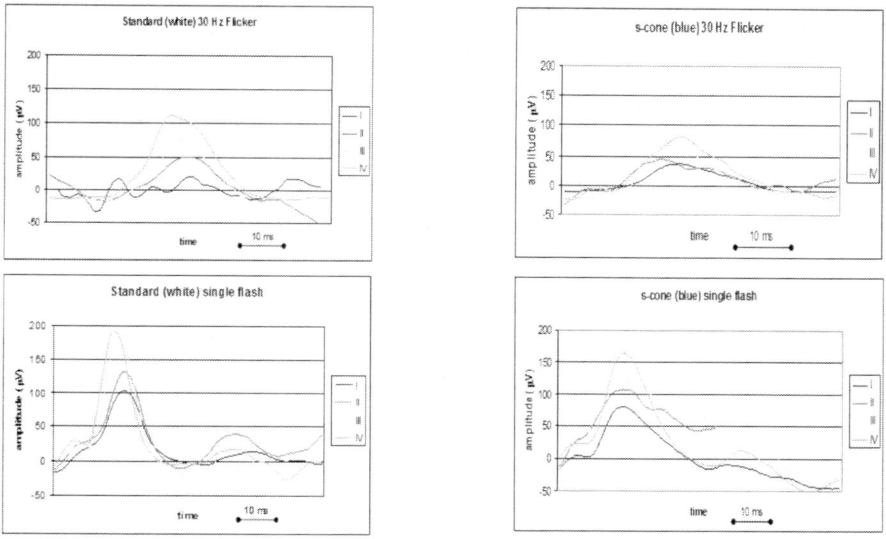

Figure 4. Typical ERG waves of the 4 groups (amplitudes near the median) The b-wave amplitudes were smaller in the preterm groups (Group I: preterm patients with stage 3 threshold ROP regressed after laser coagulation, Group II: preterm patients with stages 1 or 2 ROP regressed spontaneously, Group III: preterm patients without ROP, Group IV: age matched children born at full term) compared to controls. Graetest decrease in the amplitudes was found in laser treated preterm group. However the differences were significant only for standard single flash ERG amplitude and for S-cone single flash ERG amplitude.

Our study group wanted to investigate more in detail the earlier presumed tritan deficit by examining the cones and specially the blue cones more thoroughly. We applied standard and blue cone specific electroretinography, respectively. Under both conditions, flicker stimulation was used first, since the refractory period of rods is known to be relatively long (approximately 50 ms). Responses to 30 Hz flicker stimulus represent only the cone function, while single flash stimuli could stimulate some rods as well, even in light-adapted patients [60]. Concerning the ERG parameters, the n1 and p1 implicit times showed no differences compared to controls. We didn't find any differences between the preterm groups in the n1-p1 amplitudes either. Comparing the preterm groups (ROP stage 0-3) to control one, a significant difference was found in the b-wave amplitudes obtained under both types of standard conditions and with s-cone electroretinography using single flash light stimuli [53] (Figure 4).

Based on our results, we formed the hypothesis, that in formerly preterm children with normal posterior pole, a subtle cone dysfunction is present in childhood, long after resolution of acute phase of ROP in early adolescence. This seems to be a subtle alteration, as significant decrease can be detected only in the b-wave amplitude, but the implicit times do not differ from those of controls. We found significant reduction in b-wave amplitudes only in the laser treated group compared to controls. At the same time the GEE test showed no significant impact of the severity of ROP or laser treatment on this cone dysfunction. GEE statistics indicated a significant effect of prematurity on b-wave amplitude obtained either with standard flicker ERG or with s-cone ERG using single blue light stimuli [53].

Recent data gained with adaptive optics Fourier domain optical coherence tomography mentioned earlier, offered no evidence of loss of cones in the central retina of the subjects with ROP [41]. So in the background of the cone driven answer alteration, cellular dysfunction is more probable, than loss of cells. Previous anatomic and electrophysiological data showed lower vulnerability of cones than rods to ROP [59]. In one hand, earlier maturation may protect the cones. On the other hand, cones have twice as many mitochondria and greater aerobic ATP production what protects against metabolic insults and apoptosis [61]. Furthermore, cones, in contrast to rods, have the capability of utilizing endogenous glycogen, affording protection against the adverse effects of hypoxia and attendant hypoglycemia [62, 63]

Our findings suggested that s-cone might be affected. But as we found the same reduction of b-wave amplitudes with standard stimulation we think that m- and l-cones are also altered.

The results of the GEE statistics also support this hypothesis. As it was the degree of prematurity characterized with birth weight $\leq$1250 g and gestational age at birth $\leq$30 weeks, and not the severity of ROP or laser treatment, that could predict the long-term cone impairment. If laser treatment would be the main factor, blue cone had to show selective alteration, as they are in the biggest number in periphery [64], so destroyed by the laser ablation.

Longterm Vitreoretinal Pathologies

Although late or severe ophthalmic findings such as cataract, angle closure glaucoma, and retinal detachement re uncommon in children born preterm they interfere with function and quality of life. They usually occur in adolescence or early adulthood [65, 66].

Cataracts have been associated with untreated ROP and severe ROP 65. Michael et al. reported cases of late onset angle-closure glaucoma associated with ROP, with onset between 12 and 45 years that he thought to be caused by the shallower ACD and thicker lens regardless of AL in advanced ROP cases with significant myopia 66. In our Pentacam study we did not find any significant difference in the anterior chamber angle compared to full term control patients with a history of mild ROP, but we only examined ROP cases with stage 1-2-3 cases with favorable anatomical outcome and mainly mild hyperopic and some myopic eyes.

Retinal detachement is also a well known late consequence which can be tractional or rhegmatogenous [65, 66]. The fibrovascular tissue growing from the edge of the ancient ridge or avsacular vascular border can progressively and silently fold, exert traction and even tear or detach the retina. Abnormal viteroretinal surface and myopia also play a role in retinal tear formation in preterm patients [66, 67]. Our experiences in cocordance with the litterature showed better prognosis in rhegmatogenous then in tractional cases [67- 71].

Conclusion

In our clinical investigations with recent non-invasive assesments we demonstrated that:

- premature eyes with or without mild ROP, not only the refractive errors and anterior segment anatomy such as lens position is different and shows graeter variability, but corneal higher order aberrations are also increased compared to the eyes of term born children.
- macular structure is slightly different in preadolescents who were formerly preterm, compared with children who had been born at full term. The central retinal region is larger, and the foveal depression is decreased, due to the continuity of the inner retinal layers observed under the foveal pit. Data from OCT images indicate that the

mechanism of these changes may be impairment of the normal centrifugal movement of foveal cone nuclei and inner retinal cells during development.

- A subtle dysfunction of the cone pathways is detectable with photopic Ganzfeld ERG in the preterm subjects and it could be mainly related to the degree of prematurity. The dysfunction represented on the photopic b-waves amplitude suggests that not the cone photoreceptors themselves, but rather the inner retinal cone pathways are affected.
- rhegmatogenous retinal detachement has better prognosis in preterm born children adolescents or young adult than tractional detachement

References

[1] Darlow BA, Clemett RS, Horwood Jet al. Prospective study of New Zealand infants with birth weight less than 1500g and screened for ROP: visual oucome at age 7-8 years. *Br J ophthalmol* 1997;81:935-40.

[2] Fledelius HC. Ophthlamic changes from age of 10 to 18 years. A longitudinal study of saquels to low birth weight. II. Visula acuity. *Acta ophthalmol* 1981;2:1235-8.

[3] Abramov I, Hainlina L, Lennerise E, Brown A. (1985) Changes in visual functions of children exposed as infants to prolonged illumination. *J Am Optometric Assoc* 56: 614-9.

[4] Aiello LP, Northrup JM, Keyt BA, Takagi H, Iwamato MA Hypoxic regulation of vascular endothelial growth factor in retinal cells. *Arch Ophthalmol* 1995;113: 1538-1544.

[5] Aiello LP. Vascular endothelial growth factor and the eye. *Arch Ophthalmol* 1996;114: 1252-1254.

[6] Akula JD, Hansen RM, Martinez-Perez ME, Fulton AB. Rod photoreceptor function predicts blood vessel abnormality in retinopathy of prematurity. *Invest Ophthalmol Vis* Sci 2007;48: 4351-4359.

[7] Akula JD, Kutoba R, Hansen RM, Tzekov R, McGee D, Fulton AB. Effects of vitamin–A derivative (AG-787-14-2) on retinal function in oxygen induced retinopathy. *Invest Ophthalmol Vis Sci* 2008;49 ARVO E-abstract 2629.

[8] Connolly BP, McNamara A, Regillon CD, Tasman W, Sharma S. Visual outcomes after laser photocoagulation for threshold retinopathy of prematurity. *Ophthalmology* 1999;106: 1734-1738.

[9] Chen T, Tsai TZ, Shih YF, Yeh PT, Yang CH, Hu FCH, Lin LL, Yang CHM Long-Term Evaluation of Refractive Status and Optical Componenets in Eyes of Children born prematurely. *Invest Ophthalmol Vis Sci* 2010; 51: 6140- 6148.
[10] Cook A, White S, Batterbury M, Clark D. Ocular Growth and refractive Error Development in Premature Infants without Retinopathy of Prematurity. *Invest Ophthalmol Vis Sci* 2003; 44: 953- 960.
[11] Valenzuela EG, Kaufman LM. High Myopia Associated With Retinopathy of Prematurity Is Primarily Lenticular. *AAPOS* 2005; 9: 121-128.
[12] Quinn GE, Dobson V and Repka MX et al. Development of myopia in infants with birth weights less than 1251 g. The Cryotherapy for ROP Cooperative Group, *Ophthalmology* 1992; 99: 329–340.
[13] T. Ho, A.C.K. Cheng, S. K. Rao, S. Lau, C.K.S. Leung and D.S.C. Lam, Central corneal thickness measurements using Orbscan II, Visante, ultrasound, and Pentacam pachymetry after laser in situ keratomileusis for myopia, *J Cataract Refract Surg* 2007; 33:1177–1182.
[14] D. Chen and A.K.C. Lam, Intrasession and intersession repeatability of the Pentacam system on posterior corneal assessment in the normal human eye, *J Cataract Refract Surg* 2007;33: 448–454.
[15] ÖÖ Uçakhan, M. Özkan and A. Kanpolat, Corneal thickness measurements in normal and keratoconic eyes: Pentacam comprehensive eye scanner versus noncontact specular microscopy and ultrasound pachymetry, *J Cataract Refract Surg* 2006; 32: 970–977.
[16] J.B. Ciolino, S.S. Khachikian and M.W. Belin, Comparison of corneal thickness measurements by ultrasound and Scheimpflug photography in eyes that have undergone laser in situ keratomileusis, *Am J Ophthalmol* 2008; 145: 75–80.
[17] T. Swartz, L. Marten and M. Wang, Measuring the cornea: the latest developments in corneal topography, *Curr Opin Ophthalmol* 2007; 18: 325–333.
[18] R. Ambrósio Jr., R.S. Alonso, A. Luz and L.G. Coca Velarde, Corneal-thickness spatial profile and corneal-volume distribution: tomographic indices to detect keratoconus, *J Cataract Refract Surg* 2006; 32: 1851–1859.
[19] Konstantopoulos, P. Hossain and D.F. Anderson, Recent advances in ophthalmic anterior segment imaging: a new era for ophthalmic diagnosis? *Br J Ophthalmol* 2007; 91: 551–557.

[20] S. Emre, S. Doganay and S. Yologlu, Evaluation of anterior segment parameters in keratoconic eyes measured with the Pentacam system, *J Cataract Refract Surg* 33 2007, 33: 1708–1712.

[21] U. de Sanctis, A. Missolungi, B. Mutani, L. Richiardi and F. M. Grignolo, Reproducibility and repeatability of central corneal thickness measurement in keratoconus using the rotating Scheimpflug camera and pachymetry, *Am J Ophthalmol* 2007; 144: 712–718.

[22] W. Buehl, D. Stojanac, S. Sacu, W. Drexler and O. Findl, Comparison of three methods of measuring corneal thickness and anterior chamber depth, *Am J Ophthalmol* 2006; 142: 7–12.

[23] T. M. Rabsilber, R. Khoramnia and G. U. Auffarth, Anterior chamber measurements using Pentacam rotating Scheimpflug camera, *J Cataract Refract Surg* 2006; 32: 456–459.

[24] Hibino Y, Takahashi M, Majima A. Studies on ocular functions of cicatricial retinopathy of prematurity. Measurements of refractive elements. *Jpn jClin Ophthalmol* 1978; 32: 655-62.

[25] Donzis PB, Insler MS, Gordon RA. Corneal curvatures in premature infants. *Am J Ophthalmology* 1984; 98: 627-8.

[26] Hittner HM, Rhodes LM, McPherson Ar. Anterior segment abnormalities in cicatricial retinopathy of prematurity. *Ophthalmology* 1979; 86: 803-16.

[27] Ecsedy M, Kovacs I, Recsan Zs, Mihaltz K, Szigeti_A, Juhasz E, Nemeth J, Nagy ZZsScheimpflug Imaging for Long-Term Evaluation of Optical Components in Hungarian Children With a History of Preterm Birth. *JPOS* 2014;51(4):235-241.

[28] Saunders KJ, McCulloch DL, Shepherd AJ, Wilkinson AG. Emmetropisation following preterm birth. *Br J Ophthalmol* 2002; 86: 1035-1040.

[29] Laws D, Shaw DE, Robinson J, Jones HS, Ng YK, Fielder Ar. Retinopathy of prematurity: a prospective study: review at six months. *Eye.* 1992;6:477-483.

[30] Fielder AR, Quinn GE. Myopia of prematurity: nature, nurture, or disease? *Br J Ophthalmol.* 1997;81:2-3.

[31] Fielder Ar, Levene MI, Russel- Eggitt IM, et al. Temperature- a factor in ocular development? *Dev med Child Neurol* 1986; 28: 279-84.

[32] Fledelius HC, Greisen G. Very preterm birth and visual impairment. *Acta Opththalmol* 1993; 210 (Suppl): 63-5.

[33] Fledelius HC. Myopia of prematurity, clinical patterns. A follow-up of Danish children now aged 3-9 years. *Acta Ophthalmol* 1995; 73: 402-6.

[34] Quinn G, Dobson V, Repka M.Development of myopia in infants with birth weights less than 1251 grams. *Ophthalmology* 1992; 99: 519-23.

[35] Hendrickson AE. Primate foveal development: a microcosm of current questions in neurobiology. *Invest Ophthalmol Vis Sci.* 1994;35:3129-33.

[36] Provis JM, Sandercoe T, Hendrickson AE. Astrocytes and blood vessels define the foveal rim during primate retinal development. *Invest Ophthalmol Vis Sci.* 2000;41(10):2827-36.

[37] Fulton AB, Hansen RM, Moskowitz A, Barnaby AM. Multifocal ERG in subjects with a history of retinopathy of prematurity. *Doc Ophthalmol.* 2005; 111:7-13.

[38] Lederer DE, Joel S, Hertzmark E, Heltzer J, Mattox C, Fujimoto J. Analysis of macular volume in normal and glaucomatous eyes using optical coherence tomography. *Am J Ophthalmol.* 2003; 135: 838-43.

[39] Gürses-Özden R, Teng C, Vessani R, Zafar S, Liebmann JM, Ritch R. Macular and retinal nerve fiber layer thickness measurement reproducibility using optical coherence tomography (OCT3). *J Glaucoma.* 2004; 13(3):238-44.

[40] Ecsedy M, Szamosi A, Karkó C, Zubovics L, Varsányi B, Németh J, Récsán Zs. (2007) A comparison of macular structure imaged by optical coherence tomography in preterm and full-term children. *Invest Ophthalmol Vis Sci* 2007;48: 5207-11.

[41] Hammer D, Iftimia N, Ferguson D, Bigelow Ch, Ustun T, Barnaby M, Fultan AB. foveal fine Structure in retinopathy of prematuriy: An adaptive Optics fourier Domain Optical Coherence Tomography Study. *IOVS* 2008; 49: 2061-2070.

[42] Mintz-Hittner HA, Knight-Nanan DM, Satriano DR, Kretzer FL. A small avascular zone may be an historic mark of prematurity. *Ophthalmology;* 1999, 106:1409-1413.

[43] Yuodelis C, Hendrickson A. A qualitative and quantitative analysis of the human fovea during development. *Vision Res.* 1986, 26(6).847-55.

[44] Hendrickson A, Yuodelis C. The morphological development of the human fovea. *Ophthalmology.* 1984,91.603-12.

[45] Springer AD. New role for the primate fovea: a retinal excavation determines photoreceptor deployment and shape. *Vis Neurosci.* 1999; 16(4):629-36.

[46] Abramov I, Hainline L, Lennerise E, Brown A. Changes in visual functions of children exposed as infants to prolonged illumination. *J Am Optometric Assoc.* 1985; 56:614–619.

[47] O'Connor AR, Stephenson T, Johnson A, Tobin MJ, Moseley MJ, Ratib S, Ng Y, Fielder AR. Long-term ophthalmic outcome of low birth weight children with and without retinopathy of prematurity. *Pediatrics* 2002; 109:12-18.

[48] O'Connor AR, Fielder AR. Visual outcomes and perinatal adversity. *Seminars in Fetal and Neonatl Medicine* 2007;12:408-414.

[49] O'Connor AR, Stephenson T, Johnson A, Tobin MJ, Moseley MJ, Ratib S, Fielder AR. Visual outcome in low birth weight children. *Br J Ophthalmol* 2004; 88:1149-1153.

[50] Mcloone E, O'Keefe M, Mcloone S, Lanigan B. Long term functional and structural outcomes of laser therapy for retinopathy of prematurity. *Br J Ophthalmol* 2006; 90:754-759.

[51] Dobson V, Quinn GE, Abramov I, Hardy RJ, Tung B, Siatkowski RM, Phelps DL. Color vision measured with pseudoisochromatic plates at five and-a-half years in eyes of children from the CRYO-ROP study. *Invest Ophth Vis Sci.* 1996; 37:2467-74.

[52] Hungerford J, Stewart A, Hope P. Ocular sequel of preterm birth and their relation to ultrasound evidence of cerebral damage. *Br J Ophthalmol.* 1986;70:463–468.

[53] Ecsedy M, Varsányi B, Szigeti A, Szrnka Gy, Németh J, Récsán Zs. Assess of color vision function by electrophysiological method in children with a history of preterm birth. *Documenta Ophthalmolgica* 2011;122(3):121-8.

[54] Giusti C. Lanthony 15-Hue Desturated Test for screening of early color vision defects in uncomplicated juvenile diabetes. *Jpn J Ophthalmol.* 2001 Nov-Dec;45:607-11.

[55] Reisner DS, Hansen RM, Findl O, Petersen RA, Fulton AB. Dark-adapted thresholds in children with histories of mild retinopathy of prematurity. *Invest Ophth Vis Sci.* 1997; 38:1175-1183.

[56] Hansen RM, Fulton AB. Background adaptation in children with a history of mild retinopathy of prematurity. *Invest Ophth Vis Sci.* 2000; 46:3458-3462.

[57] Fulton AB, Hansen RM, Petersen RA, Vanderveen DK. The rod photoreceptors in retinopathy of prematurity: an electroretinographic study. *Arch ophthalmol* 2001; 119:499-505.

[58] Moskowitz A, Hansen RM, Fulton AB. Early ametropia and ROD photoreceptor function in retinopathy of prematurity. *Optom. Vis.Sci.* 2005;82: 307-17.

[59] Fulton AB, Hansen RM, Moskowitz A. The cone electroretinogram in retinopathy of prematurity. *Invest Opht Vis Sci* 2008; 49: 814-19.

[60] Marmor MF, Holder GE, Seeliger MW, Yamamoto S, International Society for Clinical Electrophysiology of Vision. Standard for clinical electroretinography (2004 update). *Doc Ophthalmol* 2004; 108:107-14.

[61] Perkins GA, Ellisman MH, Fox DA. Three-dimensional analysis of mouse rod and cone mitochondrial cristae architecture: bioenergetic and functional implications. *Mol Vis* 2003; 9:60-73.

[62] Nihira M, Anderson K, Gorin FA,Burns MS. Primate rod and cone photoreceptors may differ in glucose accessibility. *Invest Ophth Vis Sci* 1995; 36:1259-70.

[63] WellardJ, Lee D, Valter K, Stone J. Photoreceptors in the rat retina are specifically vulnerable to both hypoxia and hyperoxia. *Vis Neurosci* 2005;22:501-507.

[64] Hendrickson A e 1994. The morphologic development of human and monkey retina.In Albert DM, Jakobiec FA (Eds). *Principles and Practice of Ophthalmology: Basic Sciences.WB Saunders.* Philadelphia, pp. 561-577.

[65] Kaiser RS, Trese MT, Williams, GA, Cox MS.Adult retinopathy of prematurity. Outcomes of rhegmatogenous retinal detachments and retinal tears. *Ophthalmology* 2001; 108: 1647-1653.

[66] Machemer R. Late traction detachment in retinopathy of prematurity or ROP-like cases. *Graefe's Arch Clin Exp Ophthalmol* 1993;231: 389-394.

[67] Michael AJ, Pesin SR, Katz LJ, Tasman WS. *Management of late-onset angle-closure glaucoma associated with retinopathy of prematurity.* 1991; 98(7):1093-1098.

[68] Ferrone PJ, Harrison C, Trese MT. Lens clarity after lens sparing vitrectomy in a paediatric population. *Ophthalmology* 1997;104:273-278.

[69] Ferrone PJ, Trese MT, Williams GA, Cox MS. Good visual acuity in an adult population with marked posterior segment changes secondary to retinopathy of prematurity. *Retina* 1998;18: 335-338.

[70] Récsán Zs, Salacz Gy, Sebestyén M. *Retinal detachement in preterm born infants Hungarian Ophthalmology* 1998;135:21-26.

[71] Récsán Zs, Salacz Gy Retinal detachement in preterm born infants; adolescence and young adulthood. *Hungarian Ophthalmology* 1998;135: 29-33.

In: Retinopathy of Prematurity (ROP)
Editor: Elmira Aguilar

ISBN: 978-1-63482-644-0

Chapter 7

Intravitreal Bevacizumab In the Treatment of Retinopathy of Prematurity

Simona Delia Nicoară[1,*] and Tudor Cătălin Drugan[2,1]

[1]"Iuliu Hatieganu" University of Medicine and Pharmacy, Department of Ophthalmology, Cluj-Napoca, Romania

[2]"Iuliu Hatieganu" University of Medicine and Pharmacy, Department of Medical Informatics and Biostatistics, Cluj-Napoca, Romania

Abstract

Background: In this chapter we aim to evaluate the outcome and prognostic factors of the intravitreal administration of bevacizumab for retinopathy of prematurity (ROP), as monotherapy and associated with laser treatment, as emerged from our experience.

Methods: This is a retrospective case series that was carried out at the "Iuliu Hatieganu" University of Medicine and Pharmacy from Cluj-

* Simona Delia Nicoară: "Iuliu Hatieganu" University of Medicine and Pharmacy, Department of Ophthalmology, 8, V. Babeş str., 400012, Cluj-Napoca, Romania. E-mail: simonanicoara1@gmail.com.

[1] Tudor Cătălin Drugan: "Iuliu Hatieganu" University of Medicine and Pharmacy, Department of Medical Informatics and Biostatistics, 8, V. Babeş str., 400012, Cluj-Napoca, Romania.

Napoca, Romania. It includes all the consecutive infants who received intravitreal bevacizumab for ROP, between January 1st 2009 and December 31st 2013. The following data were recorded: birth weight, gestational age, gender, type of pregnancy (unique or multiple), timing (postmenstrual age and postnatal age at treatment), immediate result (ROP regression or progression), late ROP recurrence (52 weeks after treatment), the necessity of laser. The statistical analysis was performed with the program SPSS 22.0.

Results: The study includes 97 eyes of 49 infants. According to the number of eyes, 60 had aggressive posterior ROP (61.85%), 15 had bilateral zone I stage 3+ ROP (30.61%), one had unilateral zone I stage 3+ ROP (2.04%), 2 had bilateral stage IV A ROP (4.08%) and one had in one eye zone I stage 3+ ROP and in the fellow eye, stage IV A ROP (2.04%). One week after the bevacizumab injection, ROP regressed in 83 eyes (85.56%).

Discussion: The place of anti-VEGF treatment in ROP is emphasized. The advantages of anti-VEGF as compared to laser are discussed, but also the possible systemic and local complications associated with this therapy. The factors that influenced the outcomes of anti-VEGF treatment are analyzed according to the statistical data.

Conclusion: ROP regression rate after the intravitreal administration of bevacizumab monotherapy was 85.56% in our series.

Introduction

Bevacizumab (Avastin; Genentech Inc, San Francisco, California, US) is a full anti-VEGF human monoclonal antibody that is used off label in the retinal neovascular diseases [1, 2]. The first reports on the use of bevacizumab for the aggressive posterior form of Retinopathy of Prematurity (ROP) were published in 2007 [3, 4, 5]. The laser treatment often fails to stop the progression of aggressive posterior ROP (AP-ROP) towards retinal detachment [6, 7, 8, 9, 10]. The first retrospective case series included 18 eyes from which 17 eyes regressed following intravitreal bevacizumab [11].

BEAT-ROP (Bevacizumab Eliminates the Angiogenic Threat of Retinopathy of Prematurity) was the first prospective, controlled, randomized trial that investigated the effect of one dose of bevacizumab (0.625 mg) for stage 3+ ROP, without combining laser and bevacizumab in the same infant [12]. Intravitreal injection of bevacizumab was followed by a significantly higher regression rate of ROP in zone I as compared to laser, according to the above mentioned study. Also, the vascularization of the retina continued up to the periphery after bevacizumab, which was not the case after laser. However, the BEAT-ROP study could not address al the questions related to safety, long term outcomes and appropriate dosage [12].

We reported a 54.16% regression rate of AP-ROP following laser treatment in a previously reported case series [10]. This low regresssion rate motivated us to start using bevacizumab injections in this severe form of ROP.

In this chapter we report our experience with intravitreal bevacizumab for the treatment of ROP.

Materials. Methods

This is a retrospective case series investigating ROP regression and the outcome following the intravitreal injection of bevacizumab.

Setting

The same ophthalmologist performed all the intravitreal injections in the Departments of Neonatology and Ophthalmology belonging to the "Iuliu Hatieganu" University of Medicine and Pharmacy from Cluj-Napoca and in the Departments of Neonatology belonging to the "Saint Pantelimon" and "Polizu" Hospitals from Bucharest, Romania. The enrolement of the patients was done after the parents/tutors signed the informed consent. The study was approved by the Ethics Commitee of the "Iuliu Hatieganu" University of Medicine and Pharmacy.

Study Sample

We analized retrospectively the files of all the consecutive infants with AP-ROP and zone I stage 3+ ROP who were treated by one intravitreal bevacizumab injection, from January 1st 2009 throughout July 31st 2013.

These infants come fom a screening program in which we included all the preterm newborns who met the following criteria: gestational age (GA) less/ equal to 33 weeks, or birth weight (BW) less/equal to 1500 grams.

We also included in the screening for ROP, the premature infants with GA of more than 33 weeks and with BW of more than 1500 grams, if other risk factors were associated: prolonged oxygen administration with saturation over 93%, repeated transfusions, sepsis, necessity of more than 6 days of mechanical ventilation for the cardio-respiratory support.

ROP Classification

We classified our cases according to the ICROP revisited [13]. This is based on the ICROP classification that was elaborated in 1984 [14]. ICROP revisited considers the zone, the extension, the stage and the presence/absence of "plus" disease and adds the definition of "pre-plus" disease and of the aggressive posterior ROP (AP-ROP). AP-ROP was defined as extreme vessel dilation and tortuosity in 4 quadrants, direct arterio-venous shunting, flat neovascularization, rapid evolution, without following stage 1 to 3 progression [13].

Protocol of Injection

We used no premedication. The pupils were dilated with a mixture of tropicamide 0.5% and phenylephrine 0.5%. In order to achieve local analgesia, we placed one drop of tetracaine hydrochloride 0.5% or proparacaine hydrochloride 0.5% ophthalmic solution in the conjunctival sac of the infant, 3 times, every 2 minutes before the injection. Then we placed a sterile speculum for use in the preterm infants between the lids, we instilled one drop of povidone iodine 5% ophthalmic solution in the conjunctival sac and allowed to remain for one minute. The excess of povidone iodine was removed with a sterile cotton tip applicator from the temporal lid margin.

A nurse hold the infant's head during the procedure, the infant's eye was stabilized with a scleral depressor and a dose of 0.025 ml bevacizumab (0.625 mg) were injected in pars plicata, 1.5 - 1.75 mm away from the limbus, with a 30 G needle, perpendicularly on the globe initially and then slightly directed toward the center of the eyeball.

Following the injection, povidone iodine was again instilled in the conjunctival sac and let to act for another minute and the excess was then removed with a sterile cotton tip from the temporal lid margins. The speculum was removed from between the lids. An antibiotic (moxifloxacin 0.5%, tobramycin) was instilled for 5 days following the injection, every 8 hours.

Follow Up

The patients were re-examined the next day and then every week to monitor the regression of the disease. The follow-up continued for 60 weeks, every 2 weeks initially and then every 3 weeks, until full vascularization of the retina was observed. Full vascularization was defined as follows: vascularization as far as it would develop without an active component or clinically significant tractional elements. All the patients were followed by the pediatricians for long term systemic complications. All the intravitreal injections were carried out by the same ophthalmologist and the examinations were performed by three ophthalmologists experienced in ROP.

We considered as signs of regression, the pupil dilation, the disappearance or decrease of retinal vessel tortuosity and neovascularization, the growth of the normal retinal vessels toward the peripheral retina. The worsening of ROP was defined according to the following criteria: the persistance / reapparance of plus disease and of retinal neovascularization and the progression toward retinal detachment. In all these latter situations, conventional laser photocoagulation of the retina was carried out.

Pictures of the retina before and after bevacizumab injections were taken with a Ret Cam (Clarity Medical System, Pleasanton, California, US).

The following data were recorded: gender, GA, BW, zone and stage of ROP, other ocular findings (persistance of fetal vasculature, vitreous hemorrhage, undilated pupil), postnatal age (PNA) and postmenstrual age (PMA) at treatment, type of pregnancy (unique, multiple), complications, follow-up period.

Statistical Analysis

Statistical analysis was performed using Microsoft Excel and SPSS software (version 22.0). Data were presented as mean ± standard deviation (SD) for the quantitative variables and as absolute and relative frequencies for categorical variables. Shapiro -Wilk test for normality, Levene's test for equality of variances, ANOVA test or the non-parametric Mann -Whitney U test for equality of means were used.

Differences between the expected and the observed frequencies were assessed with the chi-square test. If the conditions for this test were not reached, the Fisher's exact test was used. P values less than 0.05 were regarded as significant.

Results

Demographic and Clinical Characteristics of the Study Sample

Our study was performed on 97 eyes with zone I stage 3+ ROP and AP-ROP belonging to 49 premature infants, treated by intravitreally injected bevacizumab (Table 1). The demographic and clinical characteristics of the premature infants are presented in Table 1.

No infant from the study sample had laser before the injection of bevacizumab. Of the 49 infants, 22 were males (44.90%) and 27, females (55.10%), 40 were coming from unique pregnancies (81.60%) and 9, from multiple pregnancies (18.40%).

The mean GA was 29.02 ± 2.08 weeks (range 24 - 34 weeks), the mean BW was 1176.41 ± 312.81 grams (range 700 - 2300 grams) (Table 1).

The ROP classification within the study sample is presented in Table 2.

Table 1. Demographic and clinical characteristics of the premature infants who received intravitreal bevacizumab as primary therapy for ROP

Characteristic	Data
Eyes (patients)	97 (49)
Male/female	22/27
Unique/multiple pregnancy	40/9
Mean GA (w)	29.02
Mean BW (g)	1176.41
Mean injection time (PMA/ PNA, wk)	35.57/6.55
Number of eyes (%) with regression after bevacizumab injection alone	83 (85.56)

Table 2. Classification of ROP in the eyes treated with intravitreal injections of bevacizumab

ROP classification	Eyes (number)	Eyes (%)
AP-ROP*	60	61.85
Stage 3 zone I with "plus"	32	32.98
Stage IV A	5	5.15

*AP-ROP = Aggressive Posterior-ROP.

Of the 49 prematures, 30 had bilateral aggressive posterior disease (AP-ROP) (61.22%), 15 had bilateral zone I stage 3 + ROP (30.61%), one had unilateral zone I stage 3 + ROP (2.04%), 2 had bilateral stage IV A ROP (4.08%) and one had in one eye zone I stage 3 + ROP and in the fellow eye, stage IV A ROP (2.04%). We noted the persistance of fetal vasculature in 12 eyes (12.37%), undilated pupil in 9 eyes (9.27%) and vitreous hemorrhage in 5 eyes (5.15%), all within the AP-ROP group.

Timing of Bevacizumab Injections

We evaluated the moment of bevacizumab injections according to two parameters: PNA and PMA at treatment. PNA at the moment of bevacizumab injection varied on our series between 4 - 12 weeks (mean 6.55 ± 1.83 weeks) (Table 1). From the 87 eyes that were treated at VPN $\leq$ 8 weeks, 73 (83.91%) had a good outcome and from the 10 eyes that were treated at VPN > 8 weeks, all had a good outcome. However, the Fisher test does not prove statistical significance ($p = 0.348$). PMA at treatment varied between 31 - 40 weeks (mean 35.57 ± 1.97 weeks) (Table 2). From the 80 eyes that were treated at VPM $\leq$ 37 weeks, 69 had a good outcome (86.25%) and from the 17 eyes that were treated after more than 37 weeks PMA, 14 had a good outcome (82.35%). According to the Fisher test, this is not a statistically significant difference ($p = 0.707$). In the eyes with AP-ROP, bevacizumab injections were performed at a mean PNA of 6.47 weeks and at a mean PMA of 34.87 weeks. In the eyes with zone I stahe 3 + ROP, bevacizumab was injected intravitreally at a mean PNA of 6.31 weeks and a mean PMA of 36.31 weeks. Regarding the mean PNA at treatment, the differences between the 2 groups are not statistically significant. However, the PMA was significantly lower in the AP-ROP group as compared to the zone I stage 3 + ROP ($p = 0.007$).

The most important data of each preterm new-born included in this study are illustrated in Table 3.

Outcomes of ROP after Intravitreal Bevacizumab Injections

One week after the bevacizumab injection, ROP regressed in 83 eyes (85.56%) (Table 1).

ROP regressed bilaterally in 39 cases (79.59%), regressed unilaterally, in 5 cases (10.20%) and progressed bilaterally, in 5 cases (10.20%).

Table 3. Data of each premature infant treated by intravitreal injections of bevacizumab

Case	Gender	GA(w)	BW(g)	ROP (OD/OS)	PNA (w)	PMA (w)	Outcome (OD/OS)
1	M	28	900	AP*/AP	8	36	good/bad
2	F	28	1000	AP/AP	5	33	good/good
3	F	32	1800	AP/AP	4	36	good/good
4	M	34	2300	3 I** / 3 I	4	38	good/good
5	F	27	995	AP/AP	7	34	good/good
6	F	30	1400	3 I / 3 I	4	34	good/good
7	M	30	1500	3 I / 3 I	4	34	good/good
8	F	32	950	IVa / IVa	6	38	good/good
9	F	26	1100	AP/AP	5	31	good/good
10	F	28	990	AP/AP	6	34	good/good
11	M	30	1650	3 I / 3 I	7	37	good/good
12	F	28	2050	3 I / 3 I	6	34	good/good
13	F	28	1050	IVa/IVa	12	40	good/good
14	F	27	1100	AP/AP	8	35	good/good
15	F	29	1140	AP/AP	8	37	good/bad
16	M	30	1200	3 I / 3 I	7	37	good/good
17	F	27	970	AP/AP	6	33	good/good
18	F	29	1000	AP/AP	6	35	good/good
19	F	28	1200	AP/AP	7	35	good/good
20	M	28	1100	AP/AP	6	34	good/good
21	F	31	1030	3 I / 3 I	5	36	good/good
22	F	31	990	3 I / 3 I	5	36	good/good
23	F	30	1100	AP/AP	6	36	good/good
24	M	28	990	AP/AP	7	35	good/good
25	M	28	1100	AP/AP	7	35	good/good
26	M	28	985	AP/AP	7	35	good/good
27	M	31	1400	AP/AP	4	35	bad/bad
28	M	32	1500	3 I / 3 I	5	37	good/good
29	M	31	1240	AP/AP	5	36	good/good
30	F	31	1499	AP/AP	7	38	bad/bad
31	M	27	1010	AP/AP	7	34	good/good
32	F	26	1100	AP/AP	8	34	bad/bad
33	M	30	1130	IVa/3 I	8	38	bad/good
34	F	27	950	AP/AP	7	34	bad/bad

Case	Gender	GA(w)	BW(g)	ROP (OD/OS)	PNA (w)	PMA (w)	Outcome (OD/OS)
35	M	27	980	AP/AP	5	32	good/good
36	M	28	975	3 I/ 3 I	8	36	good/good
37	F	27	800	AP/AP	10	37	good/good
38	M	28	1390	AP/AP	7	35	good/bad
39	M	28	1550	3 I / 3 I	8	36	good/good
40	M	28	1050	AP/AP	6	34	good/good
41	F	24	700	AP/AP	9	33	good/good
42	F	31	995	3 I	8	39	good
43	M	32	1015	AP/AP	5	37	good/good
44	F	27	990	3 I/3 I	6	33	good/good
45	M	27	1052	3 I/3 I	11	38	good/good
46	M	32	1430	3 I/3 I	5	37	bad/bad
47	F	28	730	3 I/3 I	10	38	good/good
48	M	30	1400	AP/AP	4	34	good/good
49	F	32	1200	AP/AP	7	39	good/good

*AP = Aggressive Posterior.

**3 I = stage 3 zone I.

In 13 of the 14 eyes that failed to regress after one intravitreal injection of bevacizumab, laser photocoagulation was carried out, 7 - 10 days after the intravitreal bevacizumab injection. The evolution after laser was good in all cases. None of the cases in this series progressed towards bilateral retinal detachment. The case in which laser was not possible due to the vitreous hemorrhage developed unilateral stage V ROP.

Individual Factors Associated with the Outcomes after Bevacizumab Injections

We analyzed the following individual factors in correlation with the evolution after the intravitreal injection of bevacizumab: ROP form, gender, type of pregnancy, GA and BW. Bevacizumab administered as one intravitreal injection was followed by ROP regression in 30 of the 32 eyes with zone I stage 3+ ROP (93.75%) and in 49 of the 60 eyes with AP-ROP (81.67%) (Table 3). Fischer's exact test proved that this difference is not statistically significant ($p = 0.206$).

Within the group of girls (53 eyes), ROP regressed in 46 eyes (86.79%) and within the group of boys (44 eyes), ROP regressed in 37 eyes (84.09%).

The difference between genders was not statistically significant (chi square test $p = 0.706$).

Of the 49 pregnancies, 40 were unique and 9, multiple. Within the unique pregnancies group (79 eyes), ROP regressed in 66 eyes (83.54%) and within the multiple pregnancies group (18 eyes), ROP regressed in all the 17 eyes (94.44%). The difference was not statistically significant (Fisher test $p = 0.456$).

The mean GA in the group with favourable outcome was 28.96 weeks and in the group with unfavourable outcome, 29.21 weeks. This difference is not statistically significant ($p = 0.450$ ANOVA test). The ROP regression rate in the premature infants with GA ≤ 28 weeks was not statistically significant different as compared to the regression rate in premature infants with GA > 28 weeks: 88.46% and 82.22% respectively ($p = 0.383$ chi square test).

The mean BW in the group with good outcome following intravitreal bevacizumab was 1168.37 grams and in the group with unfavorable outcome, 1237.00 grams. The difference is not statistically significant ($p = 0.450$ ANOVA test). The premature infants with BW $\leq$1000 grams did not have a statistically significant different outcome as compared to the ones with BW > 1000 grams ($p = 0.217$ chi square test).

Discussion

Natural Evolution of ROP in Correlation with the Indication for Anti-VEGF Treatment

In the normal developing retina, VEGF is released in response to the needs of the neural tissue development, ensuring the vascular growth from the optic nerve to the periphery of the retina. ROP develops in two phases: vascular obliteration caused by oxygen and vascular proliferation generated by hypoxia. Vascular Endothelial Growth Factor (VEGF) is an angiogenic cytokine that plays a key role in both phases [15].

Phase 1 is the vaso-obliterative phase and it lasts from the premature birth to at least 30 weeks PMA. After birth, the infant enters a hyperoxic environment, even without supplemental oxygen, because of the relative intrauterine hyopxia. In utero levels of PaO_2 are 30 - 35 mmHg, whereas the extrauterine levels of PaO_2 are between 55 - 80 mmHg.

Subsequently, the angiogenic factors are down regulated by hypoxia and VEGF decreases. During this phase, the administration of anti-VEGF is contraindicated. This was proved by the effects of using intravitreal bevacizumab to prevent the progression of zone 1 disease, before the development of neovascularization (stage 3 + ROP). The result was the obliteration of the normal vessels in the inner retina and the development of pigmentary dispersion in the macula with severe visual loss [16].

Phase 2 is the vaso-proliferative phase and it lasts approximately from 31 - 42 weeks PMA. In abnormal conditions, the elevated oxygen compared to the relative intrauterine hypoxia suppresses the normal demand. As consequence, the diminished oxygen tensions lead to the increase of VEGF expression [15].

The peripheral retina becomes hypoxic due to its increased size unaccompanied by the development of inner retinal vessels. This hypoxic retina becomes metabolically active and stimulates the growth of new vessels. Neovascularization occurs at the junction between the vascularized and the non-vascularized retina (traditional ROP going from stage 1-3) or in the posterior retina (a particularly severe ROP named aggresive posterior ROP). Anti-VEGF is a controversial treatment that can be used in phase 2 of ROP. The treatment is not destructive and the inner retinal vessels continue their development towards the periphery [16].

From approximately 43 weeks to at least 54 weeks PMA, there is either an advancement or a regression of ROP. In severe ROP cases, neovascularization is replaced by cicatrization and VEGF decreases. The administration of anti-VEGF in stage 4A must be very careful. In stages 4B and 5, anti-VEGF will always accelerate disease progression and therefore should be administered only immediately prior to vitrectomy. The goal of anti-VEGF preoperatively is to decrease hemorrhage and inflammation and make surgery easier [16].

Indications of Intravitreal Bevacizumab in ROP in Our Series

In a previous study, we reported AP-ROP regression rate following laser treatment of 53.84% [10]. This poor outcome and the reports in the literature showing higher regression rates of AP-ROP after intravitreal administration of bevacizumab motivated us to replace laser with intravitreal bevacizumab in AP-ROP. In zone I stage 3 + ROP we obtained good regression rates following laser (94.12%) [10]. Despite this, the much longer duration of the laser treatment and the significant visual loss associated with it motivated us to use intravitreal bevacizumab instead of laser in this circumstance too.

We injected bevacizumab intravitreally in 5 eyes with stage IV A ROP. In 4 of them (80%) the outcome was good, ROP stopped its progression towards more advanced stages. The injection of bevacizumab in stage IV A ROP must be very careful. In some stage 4A cases, with few membranes, anti-VEGF may be effective in inducing ROP regression. However, in some stage 4A cases, anti-VEGF can accelerate disease progression towards total retinal detachment [16].

Advantages of Bevacizumab over Ablative Therapies (Cryotherapy and Laser)

The Cryotherapy for ROP Cooperative Group reported a 77.8% unfavorable outcome rate using cryotherapy [17] and the Early Treatment for ROP Cooperative Group reported a 55.2% unfavorable outcome rate using laser photocoagulation in zone I disease [18]. Normally, in the very small infants the foveal avascular zone never develops. Anti-VEGF allow normal apoptosis at the macula which leads to the development of a more normal vasculature of the posterior retina [19]. This may result in better visual acuity. Intravitreal injection of bevacizumab does not require general anesthesia and it acts more rapidly than near confluent retinal laser photocoagulation. Laser does not act on the VEGF already in the vitreous, therefore ROP continues to progress for about one week after laser. Bevacizumab, even if administered after an increase in VEGF, it inhibits the molecules already in the vitreous, not only the production of new ones, such as laser [15].

Since the administration of bevacizumab allows the development of the peripheral retina, the visual field is preserved. Myopia is less than following laser ablative therapy and it is similar to the myopia in the untreated ROP cases. The factors that contribute to myopia are: prematurity itself, ROP severity, zone of the disease, treatment modality, number of treatments. Repeated laser treatments, especially for zone I ROP add to the baseline ROP myopia and myopia is more severe [16].

Characeristics of the Study Sample

We report severe ROP forms in premature infants with BW >1500 grams (5 cases) and even > 2000 grams (2 cases), which is outside the screening criteria for ROP in US.

Also, 13 of the 49 premature infants (26.53%) were born after more than 30 weeks of gestation, which is the superior limit for screening in US. Therefore, the ROP screening criteria for ROP should be adapted to each region, mainly because in developing and middle-income countries older and bigger babies can develop severe ROP and possibly oxygen-induced retinopathy [20].

Timing of Bevacizumab Injections

Because of the short window of opportunity during which treatment is effective, timing is crucial for a good outcome. We evaluated the moment of treatment according to 2 parameters: PNA and PMA. Statistical tests proved that the outcome was not significantly influenced by PMA and PNA at treatment on our series. In all the cases included in this series we performed one injection of bevacizumab. Unlike AMD and PDR, where VEGF is released continuously, in ROP there is a single burst of VEGF that promotes neovascularization. Therefore, repeat injections are unnecessary, if the intravitreal injection is administered at the right time [15].

Outcome

We registered a ROP regression rate following one bevacizumab injection of 85.56%. Regression rate was not significantly influenced by ROP form, gender, type of pregnancy, GA and BW. Regression was not obtained in all cases because VEGF is not the only growth factor upragulateed in the eye, but also other factors are involved in ROP pathogeny: insulin-like growth factor, angiopoietin-1 and angiopoietin-2 [2, 21].

Safety

We watched all the patients for local and/or systemic side effects of the bevacizumab injection.

We report 10 mild conjunctival hemorrhages that resorbed within a few days. We registered no cataract, endophthalmitis, vitreous hemorrhage and retinal detachment after intravitreal bevacizumab on our sample.

Immuno-histopathologic study proved that bevacizumab is not toxic for the immature retina [16]. We prevented intraocular infection by extreme measures used to maintain sterility. In the prematur infant, there is a large lens in a small eye. In the smallest eyes, the lens may occupy at least one third of the antero-posterior length of the eye [16]. Therefore, the injection must be performed about 2 mm posterior to the limbus and aiming posteriorly to avoid cataract and dislocation of the lens. Retinal tears and retinal detachment were avoided by using a smaller gauge and shorter length needle.

The delayed onset retinal detachment, 4 - 4.5 months after the injection, was reported following bevacizumab for ROP and it is explained by the incomplete regression of the fibro-vascular proliferation, that develops slowly into a tractional complex [22]. Subsequently, we followed all the infants in this series for 60 weeks after the intravitreal injection of bevacizumab.

We report no late retinal detachment. In the premature infants, there are some organs that are particularly susceptible to damage due to their late development: retina, brain, kidney. To date there is no study to show any systemic toxicity of bevacizumab given for ROP [16]. We did not identify any systemic complication related to bevacizumab injection in our series.

Conclusion

ROP regression rate after one intravitreal bevacizumab injection was 85.56%, with no ocular or systemic complications. The regression rate was 93.75% in infants with zone I stage 3+ ROP and 81.67% in those with AP-ROP following a single injection of bevacizumab. Even if the regression rate was higher in the group with zone I stage 3+ ROP than in the one with AP-ROP, the difference is not statistically significant.

There still are questions to be answered related to systemic effects, dosing, frequency, timing and adjunct therapies to be used with bevacizumab.

References

[1] Micieli, J., et al. (2009). A Systematic Analysis of the Off-Label Use of Bevacizumab for Severe Retinopathy of Prematurity, *Am. J. Ophthalmol.*, 148, 536–543.

[2] Lin, C.-J., et al. (2012). Effects of ranibizumab on very low birth weight infants with stage 3 retinopathy of prematurity: A preliminary report, *Taiwan Journal of Ophthalmology*, 2, 136-139.

[3] Travassos, A. and Teixeira, S. and Ferreira, P., et al. (2007). Intravitreal bevacizumab in aggressive posterior retinopathy of prematurity, *Ophthalmic Surg. Lasers Imaging*, 38, 233–237.

[4] Chung, E. J. and Kim, J. H. and Ahn, H. S., et al. (2007). Combination of laser photocoagulation and intravitreal bevacizumab (Avastin) for aggressive zone I retinopathy of prematurity, *Graefes Arch. Clin. Exp. Ophthalmol.*, 245, 1727–1730.

[5] Kusaka, S. and Shima, C. and Wada, K., et al. (2008). Efficacy of intravitreal injection of bevacizumab for severe retinopathy of prematurity: a pilot study, *Br. J. Ophthalmol.*, 92, 1450–1455.

[6] O'Keefe, M., et al. (2003). Outcomes of zone I retinopathy of prematurity, *Acta Ophthalmol. Scand.*, 81, 614-616.

[7] Récsán, Z., et al. (2003). Laser treatment of zone I prethreshold and stage 3 threshold retinopathy of prematurity. *J. Pediatr. Ophthalmol. Strabismus*, 40, 204-207.

[8] Kychental, A., et al. (2006). Zone I retinopathy of prematurity: clinical characteristics and treatment outcomes, *Retina*, 26:Suppl., S11-S15.

[9] Early Treatment for ROP Cooperative Group (2003). Revised indications for the treatment of retinopathy of prematurity: results of the early treatment for retinopathy of prematurity randomized trial, *Arch. Ophthalmol.*, 121, 1684-1694.

[10] Nicoara, S. D. and Cristian, C. and Irimescu, I. and Stefanut, A. C. and Zaharie, G. (2014). Diode Laser Photocoagulation for Retinopathy of Prematurity: Outcomes After 7 Years of Treatment. *J. Pediatr. Ophthalmol. Strabismus*, 51, 39–45.

[11] Quiroz-Mercado, H. and Martinez Castellanos, M. and Hernandez-Rojas, M., et al. (2008). Antiangiogenic therapy with intravitreal bevacizumab for retinopathy of prematurity, *Retina*, 28, S19–25.

[12] Mintz-Hittner, H. A., et al. (2011). Efficacy of intravitreal bevacizumab for stage 3+ retinopathy of prematurity, *N. Engl. J. Med.* 364, 603-615.

[13] The International Classification of Retinopathy of Prematurity revisited (2005). *Arch. Ophthalmol.*, 123, 991–999.

[14] An international classification of retinopathy of prematurity. Prepared by an international committee (1984), *Br. J. Ophthalmol.*, 68, 690–697.

[15] Micielu, J. A. and Surkont, M. and Smith, A. F. (2009). A Systematic Analysis of the Off-Label Use of Bevacizumab for Severe Retinopathy of Prematurity, *Am. J. Ophthalmol.*, 148, 536–543.

[16] Mintz-Hittner, H. A. (2012). Treatment of retinopathy of prematurity with vascular endothelial growth factor inhibitors, *Early Human Development* 88, 937–941.

[17] Cryotherapy for Retinopathy of Prematurity Cooperative Group (1990). Multicenter trial of cryotherapy for retinopathy of prematurity. Three-month outcome, *Arch. Ophthalmol.*, 108, 195–204.

[18] Early Treatment for Retinopathy of Prematurity Cooperative Group (2003). Revised indications for the treatment of retinopathy of prematurity: results of the early treatment for retinopathy of prematurity randomized trial, *Arch. Ophthalmol.*, 121, 1684–1694.

[19] Mintz-Hittner, H. A. and Knight-Nanan, D. M. and Satriano, D. R. and Kretzer, F. L. (1999). A small avascular zone may be an historic mark of prematurity, *Ophthalmology*, 106, 1409-1413.

[20] Gilbert, C. and Fielder, A. and Gordillo, L., et al. (2005). Characteristics of infants with severe retinopathy of prematurity in countries with low, moderate, and high levels of development: implications for screening programs, *Pediatrics*, 115, suppl. no. 2, 518-525.

[21] Sato, T., et al. (2011). Vitreous levels of Angiopoietin-1 and Angiopoietin-2 in eyes with Retinopathy of Prematurity, *Am. J. Ophthalmol.*, 151, 353–357.

[22] Jang, S. Y., et al. (2010). Delayed-onset retinal detachment after an intravitreal injection of ranibizumab for zone 1 plus retinopathy of prematurity, *JAAPOS*, 14, 457-459.

Index

B

C

D

E

F

G

J

K

L

M

N

O

P

Q

R

S

T